Competency Based Practical Manual for MICROBIOLOGY

Celebrating 50

Passion, Quality and Innovation in Healthcare Publishing

Competency Based Practical Manual for
MICROBIOLOGY

As per the Competency Based Curriculum (MCI)

UPASANA BHUMBLA MBBS MD (Microbiology)
Associate Professor and Infection Control Officer
Incharge, Advanced Molecular Laboratory
Department of Microbiology
Geetanjali Medical College and Hospital
Udaipur, Rajasthan, India

Forewords

Jagdish Chander
FS Mehta

JAYPEE

JAYPEE BROTHERS MEDICAL PUBLISHERS
The Health Sciences Publisher
New Delhi | London

Jaypee Brothers Medical Publishers (P) Ltd

Headquarters
Jaypee Brothers Medical Publishers (P) Ltd
EMCA House, 23/23-B
Ansari Road, Daryaganj
New Delhi 110 002, India
Landline: +91-11-23272143, +91-11-23272703
+91-11-23282021, +91-11-23245672
Email: jaypee@jaypeebrothers.com

Corporate Office
Jaypee Brothers Medical Publishers (P) Ltd
4838/24, Ansari Road, Daryaganj
New Delhi 110 002, India
Phone: +91-11-43574357
Fax: +91-11-43574314
Email: jaypee@jaypeebrothers.com

Overseas Office
J.P. Medical Ltd
83 Victoria Street, London
SW1H 0HW (UK)
Phone: +44 20 3170 8910
Fax: +44 (0)20 3008 6180
Email: info@jpmedpub.com

Website: www.jaypeebrothers.com
Website: www.jaypeedigital.com

Inquiries for bulk sales may be solicited at: jaypee@jaypeebrothers.com

Competency Based Practical Manual for Microbiology

First Edition: **2021**

ISBN: 978-81-948028-7-7

Printed at: Sterling Graphics Pvt. Ltd.

Dedicated to

My Guruji

Grandparents

Parents and my beloved Sisters

whose blessings and encouragement have always
been with me throughout my endeavor

Foreword

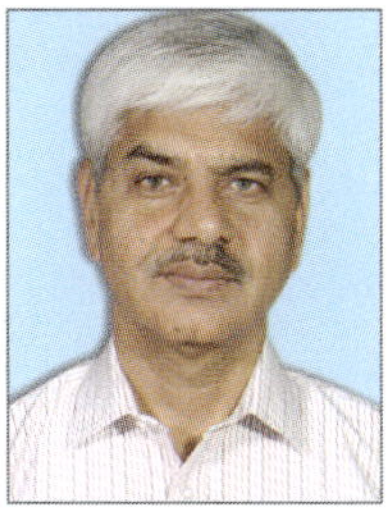

The subject of Microbiology is a rapidly changing medical field, which has now evolved to the present level in COVID-19 era, wherein it is getting more and more importance. There are rapid transformations going on in the field of all its subsidiaries like virology, mycology, immunology, bacteriology and parasitology not only in the developing world but the developed world as well. The emerging and re-emerging infectious diseases are creating havoc day-by-day concerning everyone on the planet.

Almost parallel, in recent times the Medical Council of India (MCI) has got replaced by the National Medical Commission (NMC) thereby the entire curriculum of MBBS, already undergoing a total change, has come into force this year by the Gazette notification of the Government of India. The main emphasis in the curriculum is on the latest Competency Based Medical Examination (CBME) for undergraduates MBBS and postgraduates of MD (Microbiology).

In such background, I am delighted to write the Foreword of *Competency Based Practical Manual for Microbiology* authored by Dr Upasana Bhumbla. This book is dealing with the significant practical aspects of diagnostic microbiology. She has designed the book as per the requirement and format of the new curriculum and is mainly intended for the medical undergraduates. It deals with the basic rudimentary facts, which medical, paramedical and nursing students should be familiar with in their learning process. She has used the latest nomenclature, classification and taxonomy of the microorganisms to be abreast with the current updates. Wherever required inserted the photographs for a lucid understanding on the topic under discussion. It has come out like a ready-reference in the practical fields of medical microbiology.

In this book, she has included didactic ideas and the new pattern of Competency Based Practical Microbiology, Clinical Microbiology including Hospital-associated Infections to be practiced by both undergraduates and postgraduates. It also adds up to the idea of bringing the book with many innovative chapters for learning. For theory and practical examination as well as the management of infectious diseases among the patients. Chapters range from General Microbiology, which address the basic concept in microbiology; newer concept of Applied Microbiology, very well written by her. The content of book is to make the best efforts to undergo practical training to the medical graduates and how to grasp a better understanding of the complex topics, thus, to improve the quality of diagnostic and applied microbiology.

I congratulate her for bringing this comprehensive treatise and wishes for great success for unique and relentless effort to bring forth the book for medical students as well as all her future endeavors.

Jagdish Chander
Professor and Head
Department of Microbiology
Government Medical College Hospital
Chandigarh, India

Foreword

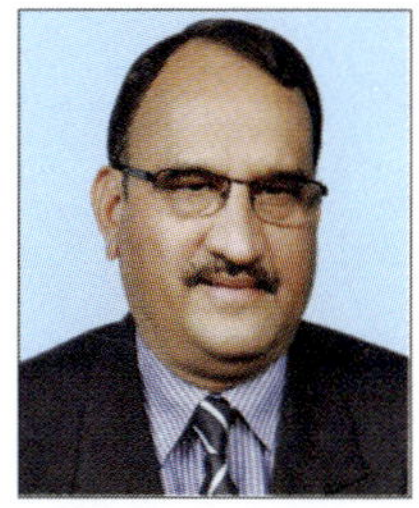

I am delighted to write the Foreword for *Competency Based Practical Manual for Clinical Microbiology* by Dr Upasana Bhumbla. Sections range from General Microbiology, Clinical Syndromes based on presentation, Recent advances, Healthcare-associated Infections (HAIs) which addresses the basic concept of Applied Microbiology, is very well-written in this book. The content of this book is to train Indian Medical Graduates and for a better understanding of complex topics. It will improve the quality of Diagnostic and Applied Microbiology.

I congratulate her for comprehensive work and best wishes for her great success. I appreciate her continuous efforts for bringing the best possible way for undergraduates to learn Medical Microbiology.

FS Mehta MBBS MS FIAS
Dean
Geetanjali Medical College and Hospital
Udaipur, Rajasthan, India

Preface

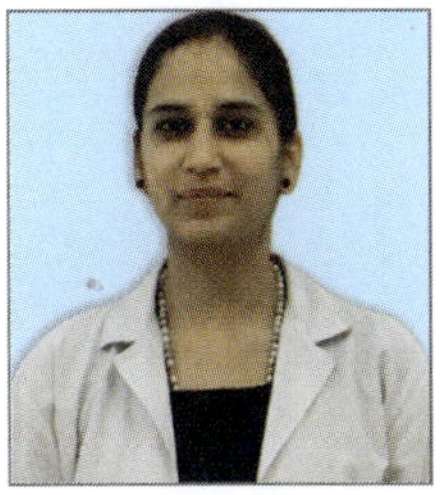

It gives me immense pleasure to present *Competency Based Practical Manual for Microbiology*. This book is compiled as per new MBBS curriculum and content of book is transformed from traditional organism based teaching to system based teaching.

This book is provided in a workbook style for Indian medical graduates for practical exercises in Microbiology. This book has been designed in a pattern to help students, learn and work on the practical and clinical aspects of Microbiology. It is divided into 8 sections which encloses 21 chapters of General Microbiology, Clinical Syndromes, Newer Advances of Immunology, Parasitology, Mycology, Virology, Healthcare-associated Infections and Applied Exercise.

I undertook this endeavor based on my experience of teaching undergraduates. For the benefit of students, the likely questions and short notes that are important in the practice of medicine have been included. This book emphasis in a workbook style so that students are able to understand and write the practical notes. The recent advances that are increasingly applied in the rapid diagnosis of infectious diseases have also been added.

Upasana Bhumbla

Acknowledgments

Acknowledgements for reviewing this manual.

Anuradha Sharma
Additional Professor, Department of Microbiology
All India Institute of Medical Sciences
Jodhpur, Rajasthan, India

AS Dalal
Professor and HOD, Department of Microbiology
Geetanjali Medical College and Hospital
Udaipur, Rajasthan, India

Balramji Omar
Additional Professor, Department of Microbiology
All India Institute of Medical Sciences
Rishikesh, Uttarakhand, India

Dinesh Raj Mathur
Dean and Professor, Department of Microbiology
Shadan Institute of Medical Sciences
Hyderabad, Telangana, India

FS Mehta
Dean and Professor, Department of Surgery
Geetanjali Medical College and Hospital
Udaipur, Rajasthan, India

Gyaneshwari
Professor, Department of Microbiology
Shadan Institute of Medical Sciences
Hyderabad, Telangana, India

Shobha Paul
Professor and HOD, Department of Microbiology
MNR Institute of Medical Sciences
Sangareddy, Hyderabad, Telangana, India

I am highly thankful to Shri Jitendar P Vij (Group Chairman), Mr Ankit Vij (Managing Director), Mr MS Mani (Group President), Dr Madhu Choudhary (Publishing Head-Education), Ms Pooja Bhandari (Production Head), Ms Sunita Katla (Executive Assistant to Group Chairman and Publishing Manager), Ms Samina Khan (Executive Assistant to Publishing Head-Education) and the whole team of M/s Jaypee Brothers Medical Publishers (P) Ltd, New Delhi, India without their cooperation, I could not have completed this project.

Department of Microbiology

Passport Size Photo

Name: --

Father's Name: --

Permanent Address: --

Telephone: --

E-mail Id: --

Registration Number: --

Date of Joining: --

Signature and Seal **Head of Department**

Competency Table

Topics	Competency	Page	Remarks
Section 1: General Microbiology			
Chapter 1: Microscopy	MI1.1	3–7	
Chapter 2: Sterilization and Disinfection	MI1.4, 1.5, SU14.1	8–13	
Chapter 3: Gram's Staining	MI1.2, MI6.2, MI6.3	14–15	
Chapter 4: Morphology of Bacteria	MI1.1, MI1.2, MI6.2, MI6.3, DR15.2	16–22	
Chapter 5: Hanging Drop Preparation	IM16.10, PE24.12	23–25	
Chapter 6: Ziehl Neelsen's Staining	MI1.2, MI6.3, IM3.14, PE34.11, CT1.10	26–31	
Chapter 7: Culture Media and Culture Methods	MI1.1	32–44	
Chapter 8: Identification of Bacteria by Biochemical Reactions	MI1.1	45–57	
Chapter 9: Principles and Uses of Antimicrobial Agents	MI1.6	58–60	
Section 2: Clinical Syndromes			
Chapter 10: Collection and Transport of Clinical Specimens for Various Clinical Syndromes	MI8.9, MI8.10, MI8.11, MI8.14, MI8.15, PE34.10	63–88	
Section 3: Immunology			
Chapter 11: Serology	MI1.8, MI8.15	91–100	
Section 4: Parasitology			
Chapter 12: Stool Examination	MI1.2, MI3.2, IM16.9, CM3.3	103–104	
Chapter 13: Morphology of Various Parasites	MI3.2, IM16.9, CM3.3	105–112	
Section 5: Mycology			
Chapter 14: Morphology of Fungi	MI1.1, MI1.2	115–122	

Competency Index

LIST OF COMPETENCIES FOR PRACTICAL MICROBIOLOGY

Name of Competency	Teaching Learning Method	Assessment	Remarks and Certificate if Required
MI1.1: Describe the different causative agents of infectious diseases	Lecture, small group discussion	Written/viva voce	
MI1.2: Perform and identify the different causative agents of infectious diseases by microscopy	DOAP session	Skill assessment	
MI1.4: Classify and describe different methods of sterilization and disinfection. Discuss the application of different methods in laboratory, in clinical and surgical practice	Lecture, small group discussion	Written/viva voce	
MI1.5: Choose and describe appropriate method of sterilization and disinfection to be used in specific situations in the laboratory, in clinical and surgical practice	Small group discussion, case discussion	Written/viva voce/OSPE	
MI1.8: Describe the mechanisms of immunity and response of host immune system to infections	Lecture	Written/viva voce	
MI2.6: Identify the causative agent of malaria and filariasis	DOAP session	Skill assessment	
MI2.7, IM6.4: Describe epidemiology, etiopathogenesis, evolution, complication, opportunistic infections, diagnosis, prevention and principles of management of HIV	Lecture, small group discussion	Written/viva voce	
MI3.7: Describe epidemiology, etiopathogenesis and discuss viral markers in the evolution of viral hepatitis. Discuss the modalities in diagnosis and prevention of viral hepatitis	Lecture, small group discussion	Written/viva voce	
MI3.8: Choose the appropriate laboratory test in the diagnosis of viral hepatitis with emphasis on viral markers	Lecture, small group discussion	Written/viva voce	
MI5.3: Identify the microbial agents causing meningitis	DOAP session	Skill assessment	
MI6.3: Identify the common etiologic agents of lower respiratory tract infections (Gram staining)	DOAP session	Skill assessment	

Name of Competency	Teaching Learning Method	Assessment	Remarks and Certificate if Required
MI7.2: Describe etiology, discuss laboratory diagnosis of sexually transmitted diseases. Recommend preventive measures	Lecture and small group discussion	Written/viva voce	
MI7.3: Describe etiology, appropriate method of specimen collection for diagnosis of UTI	Lecture and small group discussion	Written/viva voce	
MI8.15: Choose and interpret the results of laboratory tests used in diagnosis of infectious diseases	Small group discussion, case discussion	Written/viva voce/OSPE	
MI8.5: Define healthcare-associated infections (HAIs) and enumerate types. Discuss the factors that contribute to the development of HAI and methods of prevention	Lecture, small group discussion	Written/viva voce	
MI8.6: Describe the basics of infection control	Lecture, small group discussion	Written/viva voce	
MI8.7: Demonstrate infection control practices and use of personal protective equipment	DOAP session	Skill assessment	
MI8.9, MI8.10: Discuss the appropriate method of collection of samples in the performance of laboratory tests in detection of microbial agents causing infectious diseases	Lecture, small group discussion, DOAP session	Written/viva voce, skill assessment	
MI8.11: Demonstrate respect for patient samples sent to the laboratory for performance of laboratory tests in the detection of microbial agents causing infectious diseases	Lecture, small group discussion, DOAP session	Skill assessment	
MI8.14: Demonstrate confidentiality pertaining to patient identity in laboratory results	DOAP session	Skill assessment	
MI8.15: Choose and interpret the results of the laboratory tests used in diagnosis of infectious diseases	Small group discussion, case discussion	Written/viva voce, OSPE	
IM1.22: Assist and demonstrate the proper technique in collecting specimen for blood culture	DOAP session	Skill assessment	
IM3.10: Demonstrate the correct technique in a mannequin and interpret test results of a blood culture	DOAP session	Skill assessment	
IM4.19: Assist in the collection of blood and wound cultures	DOAP session	Log book documentation	
IM6.2: Define and classify HIV AIDS based on CDC criteria	Lecture, small group discussion	Written/viva voce	

Name of Competency	Teaching Learning Method	Assessment	Remarks and Certificate if Required
IM6.10: Choose and interpret appropriate diagnostic tests to diagnose and classify severity of HIV-AIDS including specific tests of HIV	Small group discussion, bedside clinic, DOAP session	Written/skill assessment	
IM17.7: Enumerate the indications and describe the findings in CSF in patients with meningitis	Small group discussion, bedside clinic	Skill assessment	
IM17.8: Demonstrate in a mannequin or equivalent the correct technique for performing a lumbar puncture	DOAP session	Skill assessment	
IM17.9: Interpret the CSF findings when presented with various parameters of CSF fluid analysis	Small group discussion, bedside clinic	Skill assessment	
PE30.21: Interpret and explain the findings in a CSF analysis	Small group discussion	Log book	
PE34.10: Discuss the various samples for demonstrating the organism in gastric aspirate, sputum, CSF, FNAC	Bed side clinics, small group discussion	Written/viva voce	
DR11.1: Describe etiology, pathogenesis, clinical fearures of dermatologic manifestations of HIV and its complications including opportunistic infections	Lecture, small group discussion	Written/viva voce	
CM14.1: Define and classify hospital waste	Lecture, small group discussion, visit to hospital	Written/viva voce	
CM14.2: Describe various methods of treatment of hospital waste	Lecture, small group discussion, visit to hospital	Written/viva voce	
CM14.3: Describe laws related to hospital waste management	Lecture, small group discussion	Written/viva voce	
SU15.1: Describe classification of hospital waste and appropriate methods of disposal	Lecture, small group discussion	Written/viva voce	

Section 1: General Microbiology

Microscopy

1

CHAPTER

COMPETENCY

MI1.2: Perform and identify the different causative agents of infectious diseases by microscopy.

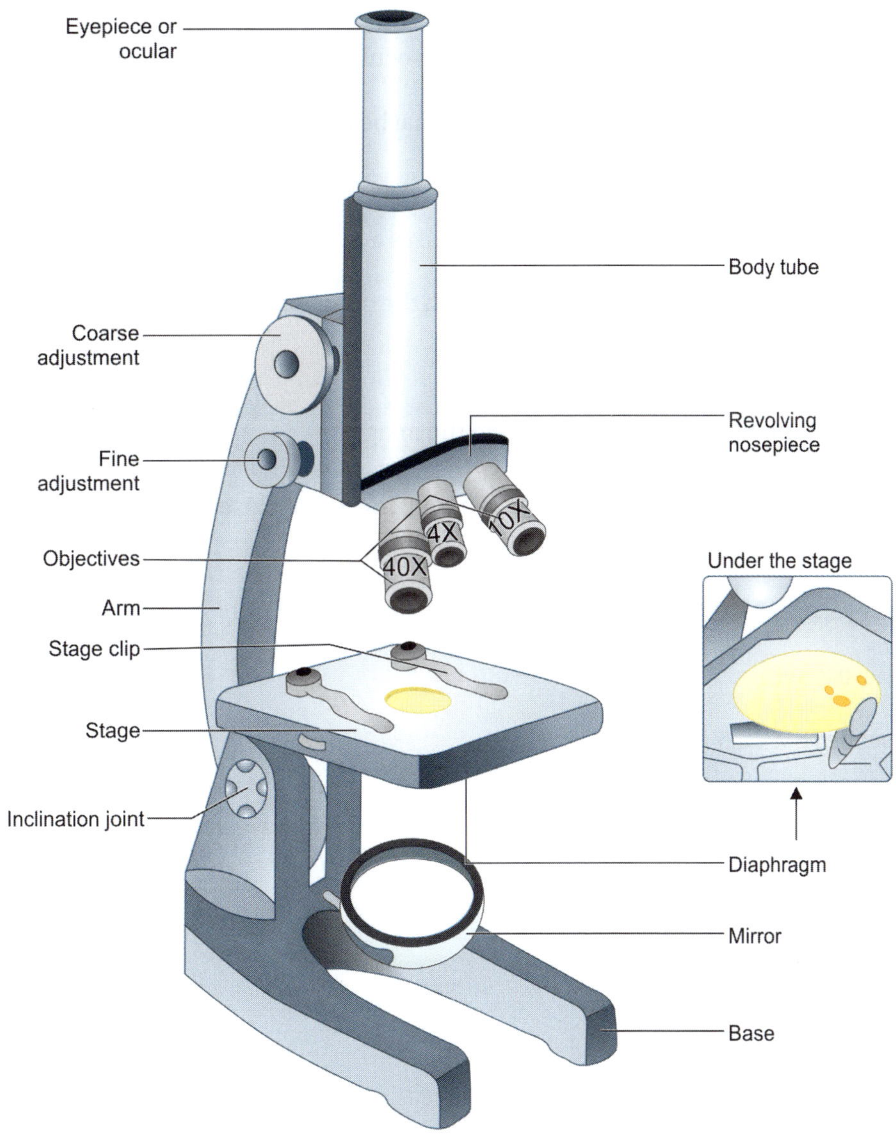

LIGHT MICROSCOPE

Principle

The rays emitted from light source pass through the iris diaphragm and fall on the specimen. Light rays passing through the specimen are gathered by the objective and a magnified image is formed.

Various Parts

- **Base:** It holds various parts of microscope, such as light source, the fine and coarse adjustment knobs.
- **C-shaped arm:** It holds microscope and it connects the ocular lens to objective lens.
- **Mechanical stage:** Arm bears a stage with stage clips to hold the slides and knobs to move the slide during viewing.
- **Ocular lens:** The arm contains an eyepiece that bears an ocular lens of 10X magnification power.
- **Objective lens:** The arm contains a revolving nosepiece that bears three to four objectives with lenses of differing magnifying power (4X, 10X, 40X, 100X).
- **Condenser:** It is mounted beneath the stage which focuses a cone of light on the slide.
- **Iris diaphragm:** It controls the light that passes through the condenser.
- **Light source:** It may be a mirror or an electric bulb.
- **Fine and coarse adjustments knobs:** They sharpen the image.

Resolution power: It refers to the ability to produce separate images of closely placed objects so that they can be distinguished as two separate entities. Resolving power of:

- Unaided human eye: 0.2 mm (200 μm)
- Light microscope: 0.2 μm
- Electron microscope (EM): 0.5 nm.

Resolution depends on refractive index of medium. Oil has higher refractive index than air.

PHASE CONTRAST MICROSCOPE

Principle

Condenser has a central opaque area with a thin transparent ring, which produces a hollow cone of light. Some light rays are bent due to variations in density and refractive index within the specimen. Undeviated rays strike a pass ring in the phase plate, while deviated rays miss the ring and pass through rest of the plate. The phase ring is constructed in such a way that the undeviated light passing through it is advanced by one-fourth of wavelength, deviated and undeviated waves will be about half wavelength out of the phase and will cancel each other when they come together to form an image.

Applications

Used for studying microbial motility, determining the shape of living cells, detecting bacterial components such as endospores and inclusion bodies which become clearly visible because they have refractive indices markedly different from that of water.

Light rays go through → condenser → specimen → phase ring → objective lens → ocular lens.

FLUORESCENT MICROSCOPE

Principle: Fluorescent dyes are exposed to UV rays, they become excited and are said to fluoresce, i.e. they convert the invisible, short wavelength rays into longer wavelength (visible light). The fluorochromes emit light of a given wavelength when excited by incident light of a different (shorter) wavelength. To view this fluorescence in the microscope, several light filtering components are needed.

Specific filters are used to isolate the excitation and emission wavelengths of a fluorochrome. A dichroic beam splitter (partial mirror) reflects shorter wavelengths of light and allows longer wavelengths to pass. A dichroic beam splitter is required because the objective acts as both a condenser lens (excitation light) and objective lens (emission light); therefore, the beam splitter isolates the emitted light from the excitation wavelength.

This epi-illumination type of light path is required to create a dark background so that the fluorescence can be easily seen. The wavelength at which a beam splitter allows the longer wavelengths to pass must be set between the excitation and emission wavelengths of any given fluorochrome so that excitation light is reflected and emission light is allowed to pass through it. A bright light source producing the correct wavelengths for excitation is also required for fluorescence microscopy, normally a mercury arc lamp.

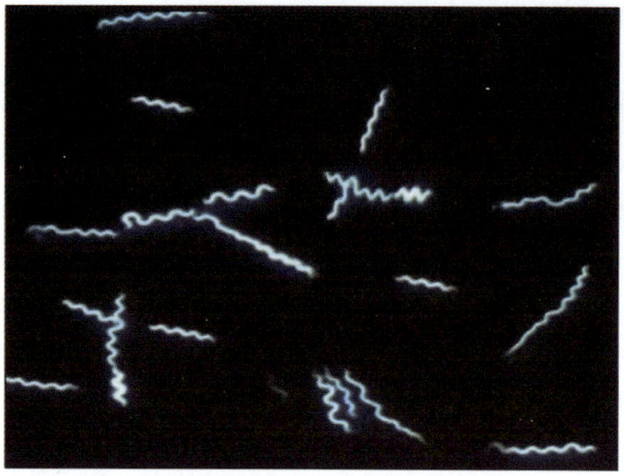

Spirochetes in dark ground microscopy

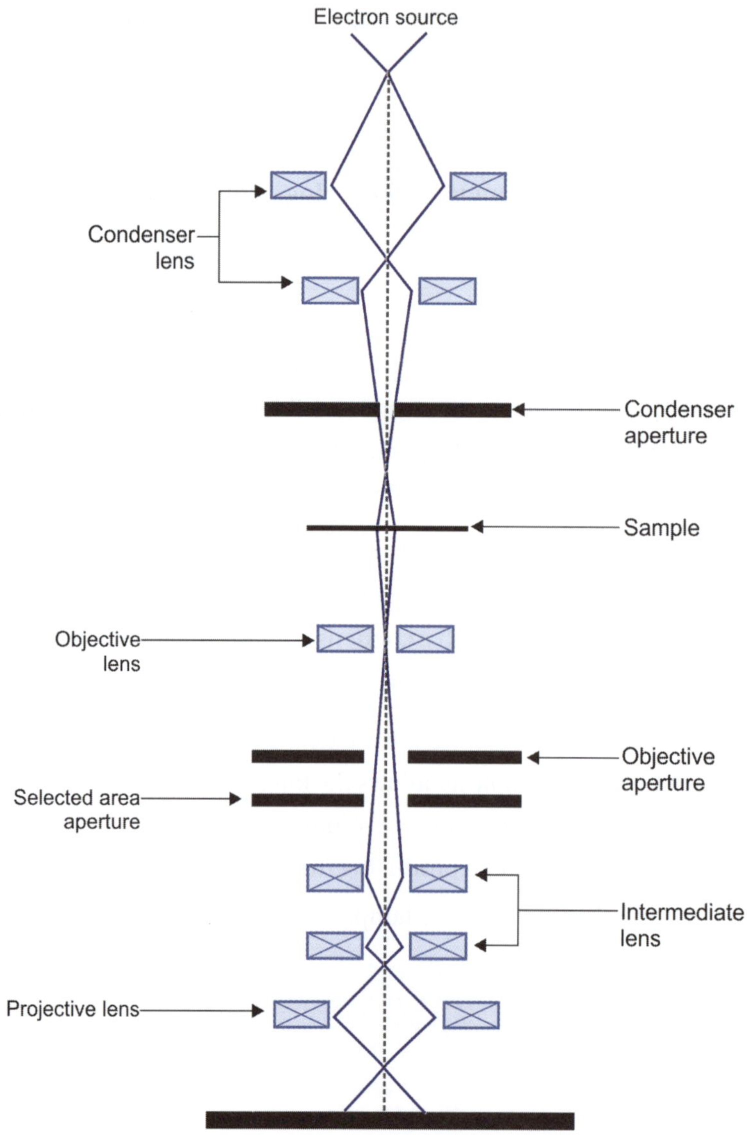

Electron microscope

COMPETENCY

DR10.2: Identify spirochete in a dark ground microscopy.

Principle

Object appears bright against a dark background, which is done by use of dark field condenser. Dark field condenser has a central opaque area that blocks light from entering the objective lens directly and has a peripheral annular hollow area which allows the light to pass through and focus on the specimen obliquely. Only the light which is reflected by the specimen enters the objective lens whereas the unreflected light does not enter the objective. As a result specimen is brightly illuminated, but the background appears dark.

Applications

Used to identify the living, unstained cells and thin bacteria like spirochetes which can be visualized by light microscopy.

ELECTRON MICROSCOPE

Discovered by Ernst Ruska in 1931. An EM uses accelerated electrons as a source of illumination.

Principle: The electron beam is focused by circular electromagnets, which are analogous to the lenses of light microscope. The object is held in the path of beam scatters the electrons and produces an image which is focused on a screen. As the wavelength of electrons used is approx. 0.005 nm, the resolving power of EM is 100,000 times than that of light microscope (0.5 nm).

Two types are:

1. Transmission electron microscope
2. Scanning electron microscope

Specimen preparation: Specimen to be viewed under EM should be able to maintain its structure when it is bombarded with electrons. Steps required are:

- **Fixation:** Cells are fixed by using glutaraldehyde or osmium tetroxide for stabilization.
- **Dehydration:** Specimen is then dehydrated with organic solvents.
- **Embedding:** Specimen embedded in plastic polymer, hardened to form a solid block.
- **Slicing:** Specimen cut in slices by an ultramicrotome knife, which is mounted with copper.

Sterilization and Disinfection

2

CHAPTER

COMPETENCY
MI1.4: Classify and describe different methods of sterilization and disinfection. Discuss the application of different methods in laboratory, in clinical and surgical practice.
MI1.5: Choose and describe appropriate method of sterilization and disinfection to be used in specific situations in the laboratory, in clinical and surgical practice.
SU14.1: Describe aseptic techniques, sterilization and disinfection.

DEFINE

- ***Sterilization:*** It is a process by which all living and dead microorganisms, including viable spores are either destroyed or removed from an article, body surface or medium.
- ***Disinfection:*** It refers to the process that destroys or removes all the pathogenic organisms but not bacterial spores. Primary action of a disinfectant is to destroy potential pathogens.
- ***Antiseptic:*** It is an agent that can be safely applied on the skin or mucous membrane to prevent infection by inhibiting the growth of bacteria.
- ***Decontamination (sanitization):*** It refers to the reduction of pathogenic microbial population to a level at which items are considered as safe to handle without protective attire.

Suffix 'cide' is used for agents which can kill microorganisms.

Suffx 'static' is used for agents that do not kill but inhibit the microbial growth.

CLASSIFY THE DIFFERENT METHODS OF STERILIZATION

A. Physical Methods

Sunlight

Heat—Dry Heat and Moist Heat

1. Dry heat

- ***Flaming:*** Items are held in flame of Bunsen burner
  - Long-time exposure till they become red hot: Inoculating wires and loops
  - Short-time exposure for fragile items like mouth of test tubes.
- ***Incineration:*** Used for disposal of biomedical waste materials. It burns the anatomical and microbiology waste by providing very high temp 870–1200°C, thereby converting the waste into ash, flu gas and heat.
- ***Hot air oven:*** Widely used method of sterilization by dry heat.

Temperature: Holding temperature of 160°C for 2 hours is required for sterilization.

Materials sterilized: Glassware such as glass syringes, petri dishes, flasks, pipettes and test tubes.

Surgical instruments such as scalpels, forceps. Chemicals life paraffin, fats, glycerol, glove powder.

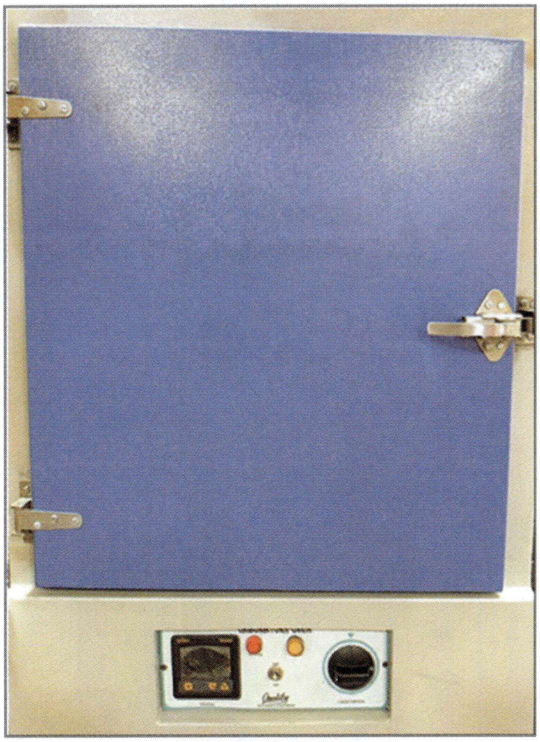

Hot air oven

2. **Moist heat**

- **At temperature below 100°C:**
  - ***Pasteurization:*** It is a method used for control of microorganisms in milk, juices and beer. Two methods are available.
    1. **Holder's method:** Milk is heated at 63°C for 30 minutes
    2. **Flash method:** Milk is heated at 72°C for 15–20 seconds followed by rapid cooling to 13°C or lower
  - ***Inspissation:*** It is a process of heating an article on 3 successive days at 80–85°C for 30 minutes by an inspissator
  - ***Vaccine bath.***
- **At temp 100°C:**
  - ***Boiling:*** Boiling of the items in water for 15 minutes can kill most of the vegetative forms but not spores. It is simple method of sterilization.
  - ***Tyndallization:*** Method uses exposure at 100°C for 20 minutes for 3 consecutive days. Used for sterilization of media containing sugars or gelatine.
  - ***Steam sterilizer:*** Used for media which are decomposed at high temperature of autoclave. Articles are kept on a perforated tray and exposed to steam at 100°C at atmospheric pressure for 90 minutes.
- **At temperature above 100°C**
  Autoclave
  - ***Principle:*** Water boils when its vapor pressure equals that of surrounding atmosphere. When atmospheric pressure is raised, boiling temperature is also raised.
  - ***Sterilization conditions:*** 121°C for 15 minutes at pressure of 15 pounds (lbs) per square inch (psi).
  - ***Uses:*** For surgical instruments, culture media, autoclavable plastic containers, plastic tubes and pipette tips, solutions, biohazardous waste.

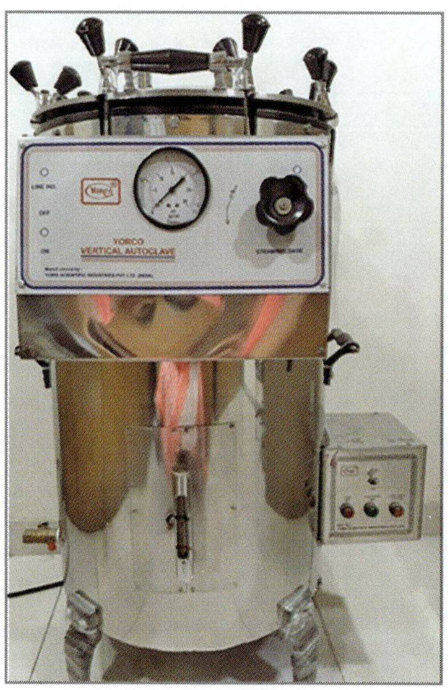

Autoclave

- ***Filtration:*** It helps remove bacteria from heat labile liquids such as sera and solutions of sugars and antibiotics. Different types of filters are:
    - ***Candle filters:*** For purification of water for drinking and industrial purpose.
    - ***Sintered glass filters:*** Prepared by heat-fusing finely powdered glass particles of graded sizes.
    - ***Membrane filters:*** Used for water purification, analysis, sterilization and sterility testing.
    - ***Air filters:*** Used to deliver bacteria free air. Two types of air filters are:
        1. **HEPA (high efficient particulate air filters)—removes 99.9% of particles size of 0.3 µm or more.**
        2. **ULPA (ultra-low particulate air filters)—removes 99.99% of dust, pollen, mold, bacteria or any airborne particle of 0.12 µm size.**
- ***Radiation:*** Two types
    1. ***Ionizing radiation:*** Includes X-rays and gamma rays. Causes breakage of DNA without temperature rise. Destroys bacterial spores and vegetative cells but not much effective against viruses.
    2. ***Non-ionizing radiation:*** Includes infrared and ultraviolet radiations. Used for disinfection of clean surfaces in OTs, laminar flow hoods and for water treatment.

B. Chemical Methods

- ***Alcohols***—are bactericidal, fungicidal and virucidal, e.g., isopropyl alcohol, ethanol.
- ***Aldehydes:***
    - Formaldehyde or formalin used for preservation of anatomical specimens, formaldehyde gas used for OTs, preparation of toxin.
    - Glutaraldehyde (2% Cidex): Disinfects objects in 20 minutes.
    - Ortho-phthalaldehyde: Used for sterilization of endoscopes, cystoscopes, mycobactericidal activity also.
- ***Phenols:*** Used as antiseptic and disinfectant, mainly tuberculocidal also. Chlorhexidine gluconate is bactericidal, sporostatic, mycobacteriostatic, virucidal and effective on yeasts and protozoa also.
- ***Halogens:*** Used as skin antiseptic such as tincture iodine and betadine. Betadine is an iodophor which is prepared by complexing iodine with organic carrier such as povidine.
- ***Oxidizing agents:*** Hydrogen peroxide, a high level disinfectant, used to disinfect ventilator, soft contact lenses, tonomter biprisms. Vaporized hydrogen peroxide is used for plasma sterilization.
    - ***Plasma sterilization:*** Plasma refers to gaseous state consisting of ions, photons and free electrons and neutral uncharged particles. These active agents present in plasma such as photons of UV rays and radicals are capable of killing microorganisms and spores efficiently.
    - ***Peracetic acid:*** Used in conjunction with hydrogen peroxide, to disinfect hemodialyzers, sterilizing endoscopes.

- ***Salts:*** Salts of heavy metals such as mercury, silver, arsenic, zinc and copper are used.
- ***Surface active agents:*** Quaternary ammonium compounds are bactericidal, highly effective against gram-positive and gram-negative compounds.
- ***Dyes:*** Aniline and acridine dyes are more active against gram positive bacteria.
- ***Gases—ethylene oxide (ETO):*** It is both microbicidal and sporicidal activity. It has large sterilizing chamber capacity. ETO is highly diffusible, penetrates areas where steam cannot reach.

Mention the method of sterilization for each of the following:

1. **Test tube**: Hot air oven

2. **Cystoscopes and endoscopes:** 2% Glutaraldehyde.

3. **Surgical dressings and linen:** Autoclave.

4. **Disposable catheters and disposable gloves:** Gamma radiation.

5. **Rubber gloves:** Autoclave.

6. **Disposable syringes:** Gamma radiation, 10% ETO.

7. **Glass syringes:** Hot air oven.

8. **Pipettes:** Hot air oven.

9. **Clinical thermometers:** Isopropyl alcohol.

10. **Basal media and Sabouraud' dextrose agar:** Autoclave.

11. **Loeffler's serum slope**: Inspissation.

12. **Lowenstein Jensen's medium:** Inspissation.

13. **Sugar media:** Filteration.

14. **Inoculation loop:** Red heat flaming.

15. **Forceps and scalpel:** Hot air oven and flaming.

16. **Antibiotic solutions**: Filtration and ionizing radiation.

17. **Vaccines:** Filtration.

18. **Dental equipment**: Autoclave and ethylene oxide (ETO).

19. **Suture material:** Autoclave and Ethylene oxide (ETO).

20. **Plastic endotracheal tubes:** 2% Glutaraldehyde, gamma radiation.

Gram's Staining

3

CHAPTER

COMPETENCY
MI1.2: Perform and identify causative agents of infectious diseases by gram staining.
MI6.2: Identify the common etiologic agents of upper respiratory tract infections (gram staining).
MI6.3: Identify the common etiologic agents of lower respiratory tract infections (gram staining).

Aim

To stain the given fixed smears by Gram's method.

Principle

Certain bacteria are stained with aniline dyes, like Gentian violet. When it is subsequently treated with a solution of iodine, mordanting action occurs. This prevents the subsequent decolorization of bacteria on treatment with acetone or alcohol. Other bacteria after similar treatment are readily decolorized and are counterstained using dilute carbol fuchsin or safranine. The theories behind it are as follows:

1. pH Theory

Cytoplasm of gram-positive bacteria is more acidic (pH 2–3), hence can retain the basic dye (pH 4–5) (crystal violet) for longer time. Iodine serves as mordant as it combines with the primary stain to form a dye-iodine complex which gets retained inside the cell.

2. Cell Wall Theory

Gram-positive cell has a thick peptidoglycan layer, which are tightly cross linked to each other. Peptidoglycan, acts as a permeability barrier preventing loss of crystal violet. Alcohol, thus shrinks the pores of thick peptidoglycan. Gram-negative cell wall is more permeable, hence allowing crystal violet to flow out easily. It is so because, the thin peptidoglycan layer in the cell wall of gram-negative is not tightly cross linked.

Presence of lipopolysaccharide layer in the cell wall of gram negative bacteria, which gets disrupted easily by the action of acetone or alcohol; thus allowing the primary stain to come out of the cytoplasm.

After mordanting with Gram's iodine, bigger dye-iodine complex is formed. After decolorization, due to more lipid content in gram-negative bacterial cell wall gets dissolved leading to formation of larger pores through which the dye-iodine complexes escape.

Magnesium Ribonucleate Theory

A compound of magnesium ribonucleate and basic protein concentrated at the cell membranes helps gram-positive bacteria to retain the primary dye. Gram-negative bacteria do not possess this substance.

Requirements

Gentian violet, Gram's iodine, alcohol/acetone, dilute carbol fuchsin/safranin, distilled water, fixed smears, compound microscope and cedar wood oil.

Procedure

- **Primary staining:** Cover the smear with Gentian violet for 1 minute. Gentian violet is a basic dye which combines with the acidic cytoplasm of bacterial cells.
- **Mordanting:**
  - Gram's iodine is a mordant. The smear is covered with Gram's iodine for 1 minute. Gram's iodine forms a dye—iodine complex.
  - The cell wall of gram positive organism is impermeable to this dye-iodine complex.
- **Decolorization:**
  - The slide is kept in slanting position.
  - Add acetone/absolute alcohol, drop by drop till the solution which comes out of the slide is almost colorless (30 seconds).
  - Gram positive organism retains primary dye (Gentian violet) while the gram negative organisms gets decolorized.
- **Counterstaining:**
  - Smear is covered with diluted carbol fuchsin/safranin for 30 seconds and wash with water.
  - Gram-positive organisms remains violet, gram-negative organisms take up the counter stain and turns pink.
- Using filter paper the slide is gently blotted to dry.
- A drop of Cedar wood oil/Liquid paraffin is placed on the smear.
- The microscope is adjusted for increased light by raising the condenser, and the slide is examined under the oil immersion objective (100X) using the plane mirror.

Morphology of Bacteria

4

CHAPTER

COMPETENCY
MI1.1: Describe the different causative agents of infectious diseases.
MI1.2: Perform and identify the different causative agents of Infectious diseases by microscopy.
MI6.2: Identify the common etiologic agents of upper respiratory tract infections (Gram staining).
MI6.3: Identify the common etiologic agents of lower respiratory tract infections (Gram staining).
DR15.2: Identify Staphylococcus on gram staining.

Staphylococci

- Gram-positive cocci arranged in clusters, short chains, as the cell division occurs in all the plane.
- They are 1 μm in size. Catalase positive, coagulase positive.
- Various toxins produced are hemolysins, leukocidins, exfoliative toxin, enterotoxin, toxic shock syndrome toxin.
- Causes skin and soft tissue infections such as follicultis, furuncle, carbuncle, pyomyositis, abscess, respiratory tract infections such as VAP, pneumothorax, bacteremia, urinary tract infection (UTI), food poisoning.

COMPETENCY

MI2.3: Identify the microbial agents causing rheumatic heart disease and infective endocarditis.

Streptococci

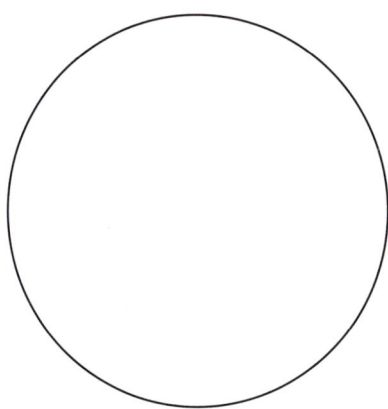

- Gram-positive cocci arranged in long chains, 0.5–1 μm.
- Toxins involved are hemolysins, streptolysin O and S, streptococcal pyrogenic toxin and enzymes such as streptokinase, streptodornase, hyaluronidase, NADase, serum opacity factor.
- Causes sore throat, pharyngitis, scarlet fever, impetigo, cellulitis, erysipelas, necrotising fasciitis.
- Nonsuppurative complications such as rheumatic fever and acute glomerulonephritis.

Pneumococci

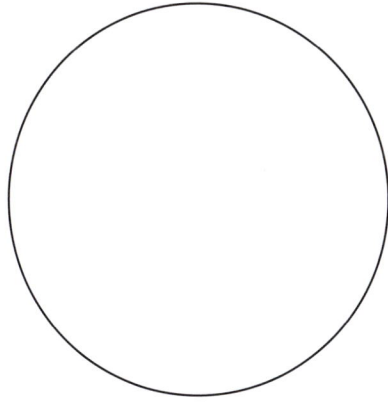

- Gram-positive diplococci, lanceolate shaped.
- Virulence factor is capsular polysaccharide.
- Causes lobar pneumonia, empyema and invasive pneumococcal disease.
- Bile soluble and Optochin sensitive.

Enterococcus

- Gram-positive oval shaped diplococci (spectacle shaped).
- *E. faecium* and *E. faecalis* are important species.
- Catalase negative and bile esculin is positive.
- Cases UTI, bacteremia, endocarditis, intra-abdominal pelvic and soft tissue infections, sepsis.
- Hospital acquired organism leading to HAIs.

Actinomyces

- Gram-positive filamentous bacteria.
- Filamentous forming mycelia structure such as fungi.
- On BHI agar—forms spidery colonies at 48 hours.
- Common cause of dental infections, brain abscess, soft tissue infections, bone destruction.

Neisseria Meningitidis (Meningococcus)

- Gram-negative diplococci with adjacent ends flattened (half moon shaped).
- Capsular polysaccharide.
- Causes pyogenic meningitis, chronic meningococcemia, septicemia and rarely Waterhouse-Friderichsen syndrome.

Neisseria Gonorrhoeae (Gonococcus)

- Gram-negative diplococci, intracellular organism.
- Bean-shaped/kidney-shaped with concave adjacent sides.
- Causes sexually transmitted diseases such as gonorrhoea.

Escherichia Coli/Family (Enterobacteriaceae)

- Gram-negative bacilli, aerobes and facultative anaerobes, non-fastidious, can grow on ordinary media.
- Catalase positive, oxidase negative.
- Ferments glucose to produce acid with or without gas.
- Reduce nitrates to nitrites.
- Mainly causes UTI and diarrhea.

COMPETENCY

DR10.2: Identify spirochete in a dark ground microscopy.

Treponema Pallidum

- *T. pallidum* is a spirochete.
- 6–14 μm in size with 6–12 spirals.
- Rigid spiral forms which is actively motile, seen under dark ground microscope.
- Possess endoflagella, responsible for motility such as Flexion-extension type, corkscrew type rotatory movement, translatory type.
- Causes sexually transmitted disease: Syphilis.

COMPETENCY

IM3.14, 4.13: Perform and interpret a sputum Gram stain.

Practical 1

Stain the given smear by Gram's technique and record your finding with a suitable diagram.	Stain the given smear by Gram's technique and record your finding with a suitable diagram.
Observation (In terms of: Color, Gram reaction, shape, arrangement).	**Observation (In terms of: Color, Gram reaction, shape, arrangement).**
Inference:	**Inference:**

Practical 2

Stain the given smear by Gram's technique and record your finding with a suitable diagram.	**Stain the given smear by Gram's technique and record your finding with a suitable diagram.**
Observation (In terms of: Color, Gram reaction, shape, arrangement).	**Observation (In terms of: Color, Gram reaction, shape, arrangement).**
Inference:	**Inference:**

Hanging Drop Preparation

5

CHAPTER

COMPETENCY
PE24.12: Perform and interpret stool examination including hanging drop.
IM16.10: Identify Vibrio cholerae in a hanging drop specimen.

Aim

To study the morphology and motility of bacteria in the given suspension.

Requirements

A cavity slide, coverslip, vaseline, microscope and the bacterial suspension to be examined.

Procedure

- Vaseline is applied to the four corners of a clean coverslip.
- Using a sterile loop, a loopful of the given suspension is placed on the center of the coverslip.
- A cavity slide is inverted over the cover slip so that the drop of suspension is in the center of the cavity.
- The slide is quickly and carefully turned over so that the coverslip is on the top with the drop hanging into the cavity.
- The microscope is adjusted for reduced light by lowering the condenser, and using the concave mirror.
- The edge of the drop is focussed under low power. The microscope is then turned to high power to observe the morphology and motility of the bacteria in the given suspension.

Practical 1

Prepare a hanging drop of the given suspension, and record your findings with a suitable diagram.

Observation

a. **Shape:**

b. **Motility:**

Inference:

Q1. HOW WILL YOU DIFFERENTIATE TRUE MOTILITY FROM BROWNIAN/MOVEMENT? WHAT ARE THE DIFFERENT TYPE OF MOTILITY?

Q2. MENTION

a. **Some motile bacteria:**

b. **Some nonmotile bacteria:**

c. **Some bacteria that is nonmotile at 37°C, but motile at 22°C:**

Q3. WHEN DO MOTILE ORGANISMS BECOME NONMOTILE?

Ziehl-Neelsen's Staining

6
CHAPTER

COMPETENCY
MI1.2: Perform and identify the different causative agents of Infectious diseases by microscopy.
MI6.3: Identify the common etiologic agents of lower respiratory tract infections.
IM3.14, 4.14; PE 34.11; CT1.10: Perform and interpret a sputum Acid-fast bacilli (AFB) stain.

Aim: To stain the given fixed smear of sputum by Ziehl-Neelsen's technique for detection of *Mycobacterium*.

Principle: Aniline dye solutions do not readily penetrate the substance of the tubercle bacilli because of presence of mycolic acid in cell wall; therefore it is not suitable for staining. With strong staining solution that contains phenol and with the application of heat, which act as a mordant, it can be made to penetrate the bacillus. Once stained the tubercle bacillus will withstand the action of powerful decolorizing agents, thus retaining the stain.

Requirements: Strong carbol fuchsin, 20–25% H_2SO_4, 95% alcohol or acid alcohol, methylene blue solution, distilled water, spirit lamp, compound microscope and cedar wood oil/liquid paraffin.

Composition of Strong Carbol Fuchsin

Basic fuchsin	: 5 g
Absolute alcohol	: 50 mL
Phenol (crystalline)	: 25 g
Distilled water	: 500 mL

Procedure

Primary Staining and Mordanting

The fixed smear is flooded with strong Carbol fuchsin for 5 minute and heated intermittently. Until the steam rises, taking care to see that the stain does not boil and smear does not get charred. Smear is then washed well with distilled water. The basic fuchsin in strong carbol fuchsin is a basic stain, while carbolic acid acts as a mordant. On heating, the mycolic acid in the cell wall of the acid fast organisms is liquefied and the basic stain imbibed by the organism is fixed by the mordant.

Decolorization

The slide is then covered with 20–25% H_2SO_4 for 2–3 mins and washed with water. This step is repeated till the smear becomes colorless. With this, only acid fast organisms retain the basic stain, while the cells and other organisms are rendered colorless.

Decolorize it with 95% alcohol or acid alcohol. Decolorizing with alcohol; saprophytes can be differentiated from *Mycobacterium tuberculosis*, as saprophytes are only acid fast whereas *Mycobacterium* tubercle bacilli is acid as well as alcohol fast.

Counterstaining

- The slide is covered with Methylene blue for 1–2 mins, washed with water and blotted to dry.
- Acid fast organisms remain red while the other organisms and cells, take up the counter stain and turn blue.
- A drop of cedar wood oil or liquid paraffin is placed on the stained smear.
- The microscope is adjusted for increased light by raising the condenser and smear is examined under the oil immersion objective.

RNTCP GRADING/NATIONAL TUBERCULOSIS ELIMINATION PROGRAMME (NTEP)

Ziehl-Neelsen Staining Grading			
Finding	*No. of fields*	*Grading*	*Result*
No AFB in 100 oil immersion field	100	0	Neg
1-9 AFB per 100 oil immersion field	100	scanty	Pos
10–99 AFB per 100 oil immersion fields	100	1+	Pos
1-10 AFB per oil immersion field	50	2+	Pos
>10 AFB per oil immersion field	20	3+	Pos

Stain the given smear of sputum by Ziehl-Nelsen's technique and record your findings with a suitable diagram.

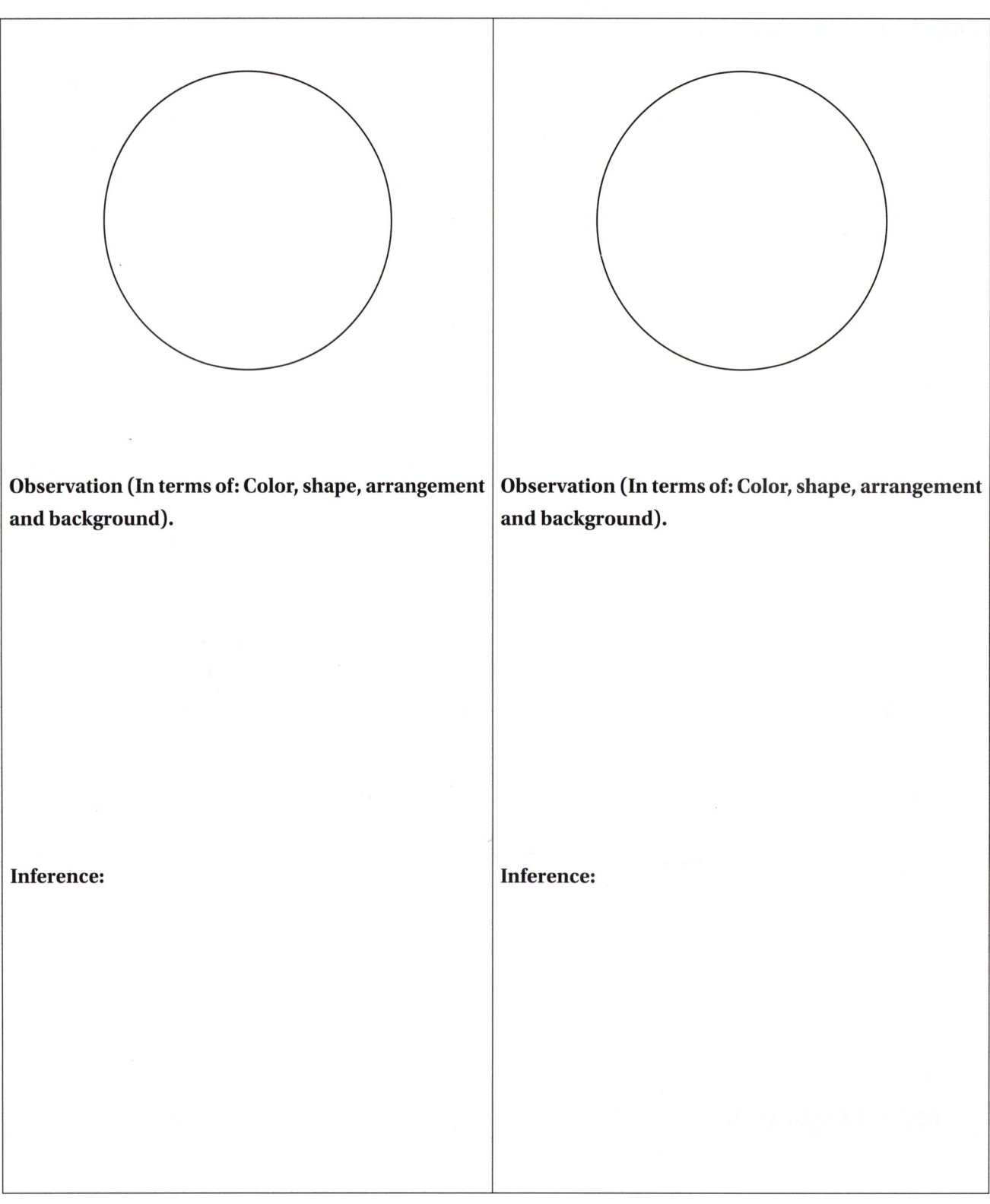

Observation (In terms of: Color, shape, arrangement and background).	**Observation (In terms of: Color, shape, arrangement and background).**
Inference:	**Inference:**

COMPETENCY

CT1.7: Perform and interpret PPD (Mantoux) and describe and discuss indications.

IM4.20: Interpret a PPD (Mantoux). PE 34.7: Interpret a Mantoux test.

MANTOUX TEST

Principle: Tuberculin skin test is the classic clinical demonstration of the function of the delayed-type hypersensitivity response. When an antigen, i.e. purified protein derivative (PPD) of tubercle bacilli is injected intradermally in an individual, immune response of person who has been exposed to the bacteria is expected to mount within 48–72 hours, leading to the formation of **induration** (a raised bump in the area of injection) which is due to the influx and activation of macrophages.

Test Procedure

Inject a standard dose of five tuberculin units (1TU) (0.1 mL) intradermally into flexor aspect of forearm (into the skin) using 28 or 26-gauge needle or tuberculin syringe from which 0.1 mL can be delivered accurately. The fluid makes a little bump (wheal) under the skin. A circle may be drawn around the test area with a pen. Results should be read 48 to 72 hours later.

Reading the results: The skin test reaction should be read between 48 and 72 hours after administration. At the site of inoculation, an induration surrounded by erythema is produced. Width of induration is:
- ≥10 mm: Positive (tuberculin reactors)
- 6–9 mm: Equivocal/doubtful reaction
- <5 mm: Negative reaction.

Interpretation of Results

Adults: Positive tests indicate present or past exposure of tubercle bacilli but not confirm the presence of active stage of disease.
Children: Positive test indicates active infection and is used as a diagnostic marker.
False-positive: Test becomes positive after BCG vaccination and non-tuberculous mycobacteria infection.
False-negative: In early or advanced TB, military TB, decreased immunity.

Mantoux Test

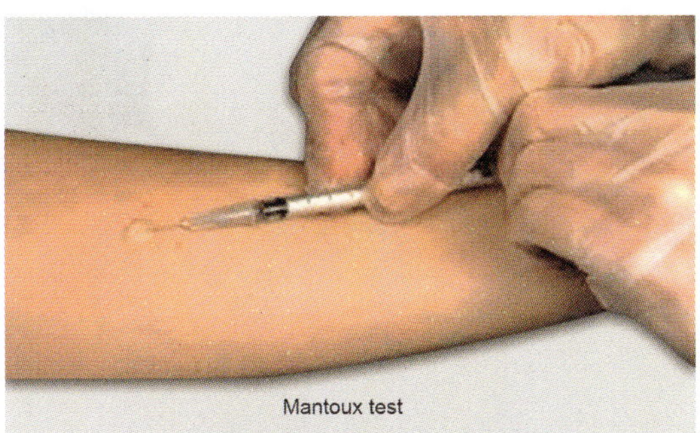

0.1 mL PPD containing 1TU

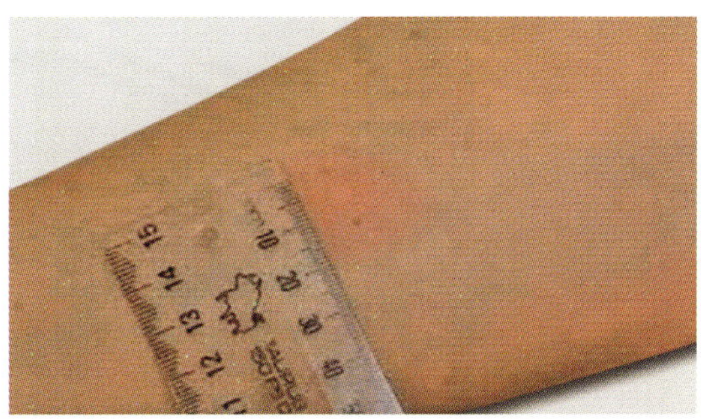

Positive test – Induration >10 mm

COMPETENCY

PE 34.6: Identify a BCG scar.

CT 1.13: Describe and discuss the origins, indications, technique of administration, efficacy and complications of BCG vaccine.

Bacillus Calmette-Guerin (BCG) vaccine is live attenuated vaccine, is strain of *M. bovis* attenuated by 239 serial subcultures in a glycerine-bile-potato-medium over a period of 13 years. Immunity may last for 10–15 years.

- Dose and strength: 0.1 mL containing 0.1 mg TU
- Administered at birth as per Universal Immunisation Programme
- Alcohol is not be used to wipe the skin
- Site: Above the insertion of left deltoid
- Route: Intradermal route by using 26 gauge tuberculin syringe.

Phenomena after BCG

- **After 2–3 weeks:** Papule develops
- **5-6 weeks:** Shallow ulcer, covered with crust
- **6-12 weeks:** Permanent tiny scar (4–8 mm diameter).

Complications

- **Local:** Abscess, indolent ulcer, keloid, confluent lesions, lupoid lesions
- **Regional:** Enlargement and suppuration of draining lymph nodes
- **General:** Fever, mediastinal adenitis, erythema nodosum.

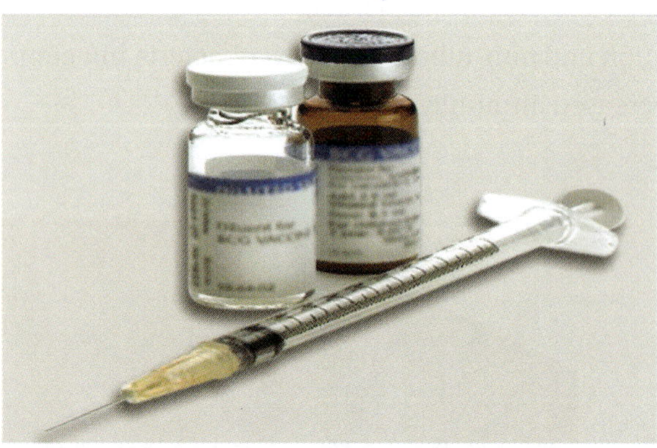

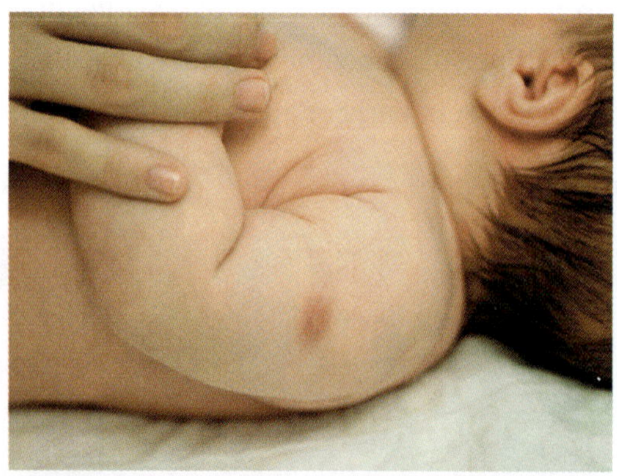

Q1. WHAT ARE THE DIFFERENCES BETWEEN *MYCOBACTERIUM TUBERCULOSIS* AND *MYCOBACTERIUM LEPRAE*?

		Mycobacterium tuberculosis	*Mycobacterium leprae*
a. Morphology	:		
b. Staining technique	:		
c. Generation time	:		
d. Culture	:		
e. Laboratory animals used	:		

Q2. WHAT ARE THE VARIOUS CONCENTRATIONS OF H_2SO_4 USED FOR VARIOUS MYCOBACTERIA?

Q3. WHAT IS KINYOUN STAINING?

Culture Media and Culture Methods

7

CHAPTER

COMPETENCY

MI1.1: Describe the different causative agents of Infectious diseases, methods used in their detection and discuss the role of microbes in health and disease.

Definition

Culture media are required to grow the organism from the infected material to identify the causative pathogen for their antibiotic susceptibility test. Basic constituents of solid culture media are:

- Water : Source of hydrogen and oxygen
- Electrolyte : Sodium chloride or other electrolytes
- Peptone : Complex mixture of partially digested proteins
- Meat extract : Contains protein degradation products, inorganic salts, carbohydrates and growth factors
- **Agar-agar : Prepared from sea weed (algae-gelidium spp.). Used in conc. of 2–3%. It melts at 98°C and solidifies at 42°C. It is an inert substance, neither stimulate nor it inherit the growth.**
- Blood or serum : Used for enriching culture media. 5–10% sheep blood is used for enriched media to provide extra nutrition to fastidious organisms.

Classification of Media

1. Based on Physical State

- Liquid media
- Semi-solid media
- Solid media

2. Based on Presence of Molecular Oxygen and Reducing Substances

- Aerobic media
- Anaerobic media

3. Based on Nutritional Factors

- Simple media
- Complex media
- Synthetic media
- Special media
  - Enriched media
  - Enrichment media
  - Selective media
  - Differential media
  - Indicator media
  - Transport media

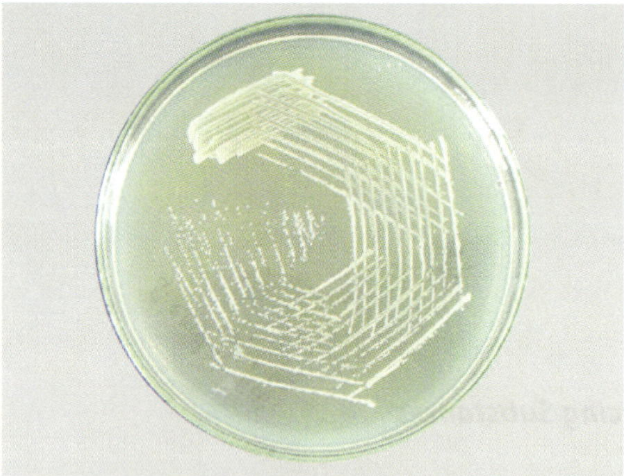

Nutrient agar

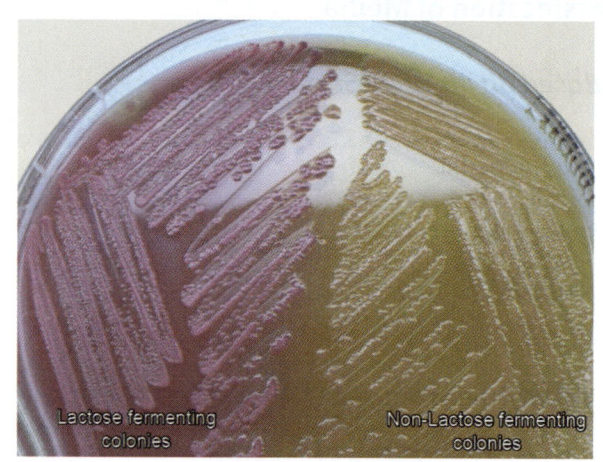

MacConkey's agar

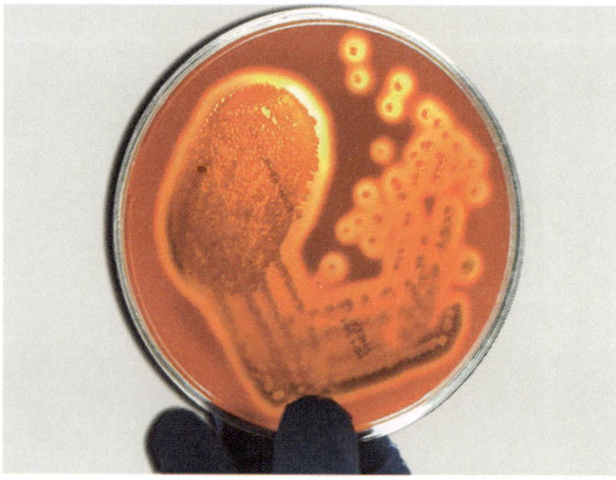

Blood agar

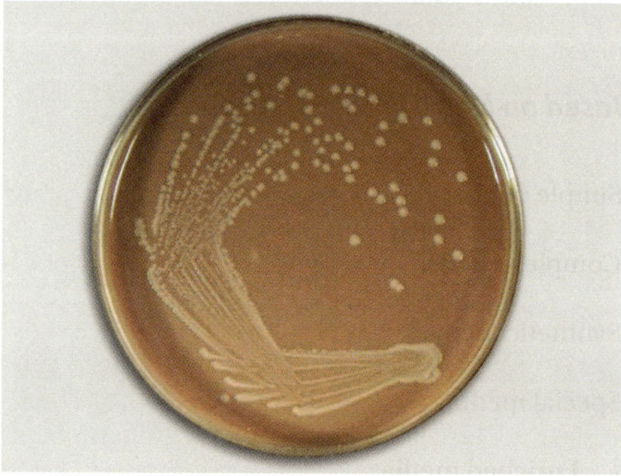

Chocolate agar

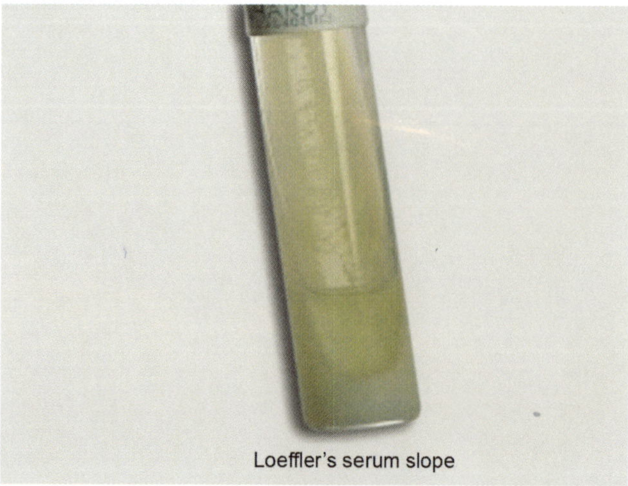

Loffler's serum slope

I. CULTIVATION OF AEROBIC BACTERIA

Culture Media (Aerobic)

Solid Media: Dispensed in petri dishes/McCartney bottles.

TYPE OF MEDIUM	NAME OF MEDIUM	COMPOSITION	LABORATORY USE
A. Simple	***Nutrient agar***	Peptone + Meat extract + Agar + NaCl	Culture and demonstration of pigmentation of different bacteria
B. Complex/Special **a. Differential**	***MacConkey's agar***	Lactose + Peptone + NaCl + Bile salts + Neutral red + Agar	Differentiate between lactose and non-lactose fermenters
b. Enriched	***1. Blood agar***	Nutrient agar + 5% Sheep blood	Differentiate between hemolytic and non-hemolytic bacteria
	2. Chocolate agar	Blood agar heated at 75°C for 10–15 mins leads to release of X and V factors	*H. influenzae, Neisseria*
	3. Loeffler's serum slope	Nutrient broth + glucose + horse serum	*Corynebacterium diphtheriae*

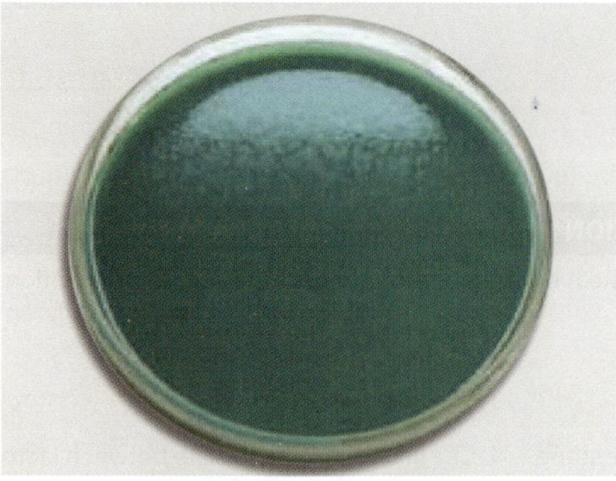

Wilson and Blair medium

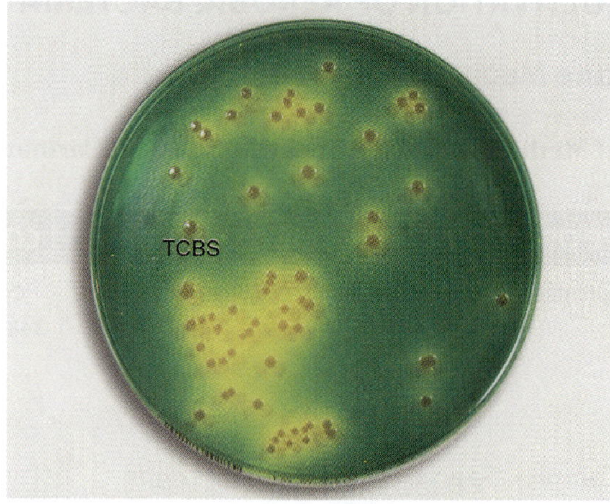

TCBS medium

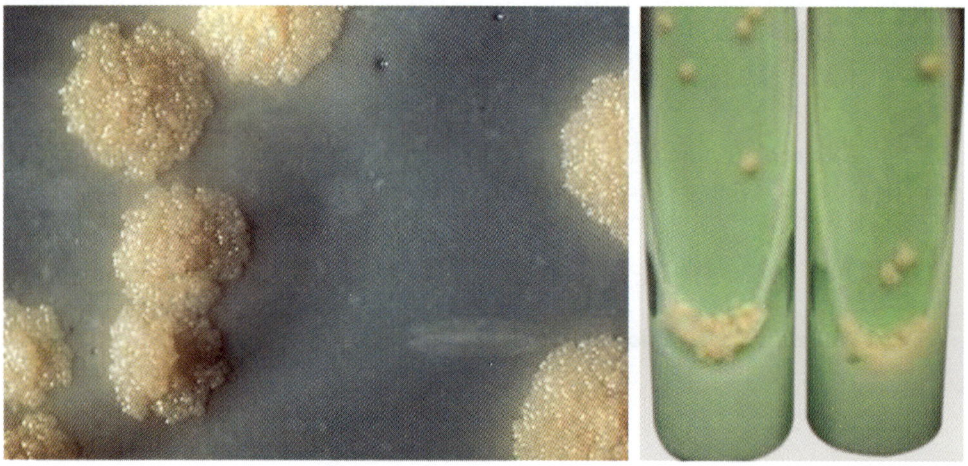

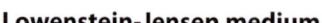

Lowenstein-Jensen medium

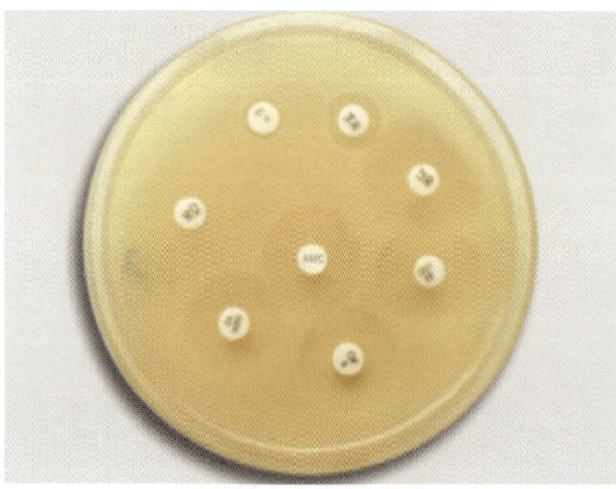

Mueller-Hinton agar

Contd...

TYPE OF MEDIUM	NAME OF MEDIUM	COMPOSITION	LABORATORY USE
c. Selective	***1. Thayer-Martin mediun***	Agar base + Hb + growth factor + antibiotics like Vancomycin, Colistin + Nystatin	Isolation of *Neisseria gonorrhoeae*
	2. Pottassium tellurite agar	Blood agar + potassium tellurite	For *Corynebacterium diphtheriae*
	3. Wilson and Blair medium	Nutrient agar + glucose phosphate + brilliant green + bismuth sulphate	Isolation of *Salmonella* spp.
	4. Deoxycholate citrate agar (DCA)	Peptone + Lactose + Sodium deoxycholate + sodium citrate+ neutral red	Isolation of *Salmonella* and Shigella
	5. TCBS medium (thiosulphate citrate bile salt sucrose agar)	Peptone+ sodium thiosulphate+ sodium citrate + NaCl + sucrose + ox bile + bromothymol blue	Isolation of *Vibrio cholerae*
	6. Lowenstein-Jensen medium	Egg + glycerol + NaCl + malachite green	Isolation of *mycobacteria* tubercle
	7. Mueller-Hinton agar	Beef extract + casein hydrosylate + starch	For antibiotic susceptibility testing

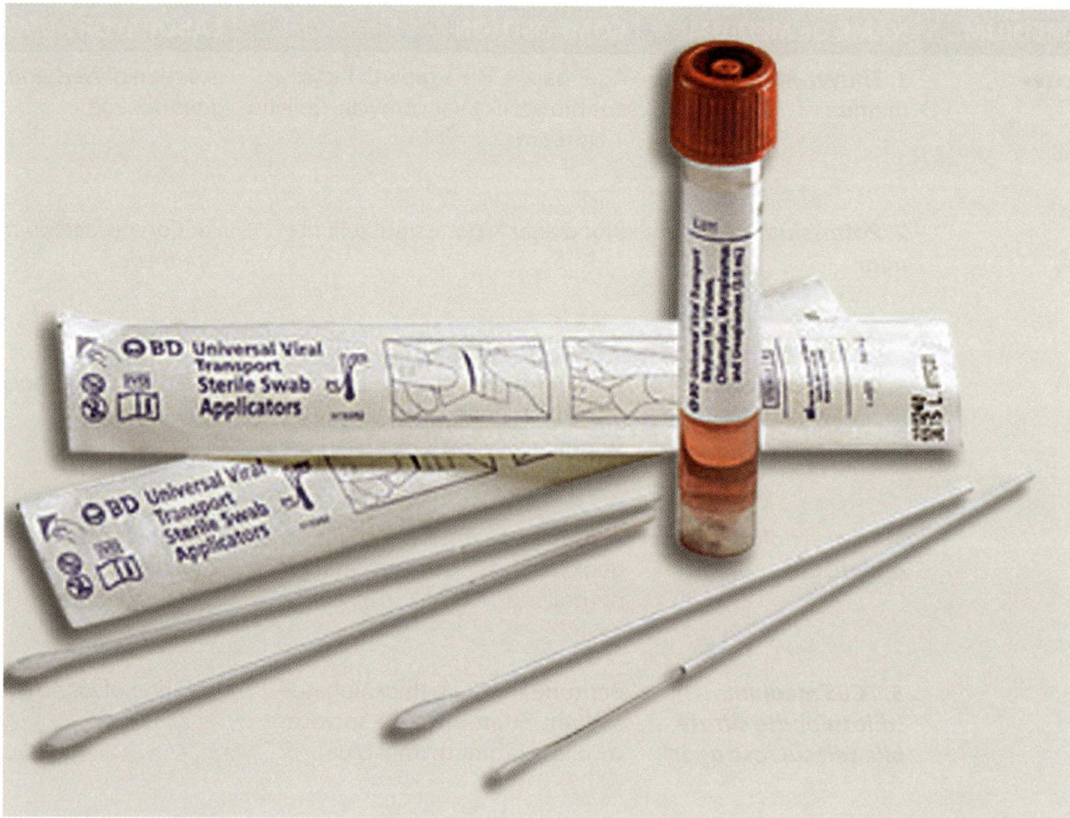

Viral transport medium

Transport media: It is devised to maintain the viability of a pathogen and to avoid overgrowth of other containments during transit of sample from patient to laboratory. It is available as sterile disposable swab kits.

NAME OF THE MEDIUM	COMPOSITION	LABORATORY USE
Stuart transport medium	Sodium thioglycolate + sodium glycerophosphate + calcium chloride + agar + methylene blue + distilled water	For maintaining the viability of *Neisseria gonococci* on swab
Amie's transport medium	Sodium thioglycolate + NaCl+ KCl + $CaCl_2$ + disodium hydrogen phosphate + potassium dihydrogn phosphate + charcoal + agar + distilled water	For maintaining the viability of *Neisseria gonococci* on swab
Pike's medium	Blood agar containing crystal violet + sodium azide	For *Strep. pyogenes, H. influenzae* swabs
Glycerol saline transport medium	Glycerol + NaCl + disodium hydrogen phosphate + phenol red 0.02% + water	For *Salmonella typhi* feaces culture
Venkat Ramakrishna medium	Crude sea salt + peptone + distilled water at pH- 8.6–8.9	For *Vibrio cholerae*
Viral transport medium (VTM)	Modified Hank's Balanced Salt Solution supplemented with bovine serum albumin, sucrose, glutamic acid, and gelatin.	For transporting H1N1, Novel coronavirus (nCOVID) samples

Liquid Media: Dispensed in tubes.

TYPE OF MEDIUM	NAME OF MEDIUM	COMPOSITION	LABORATORY USE
A. Basal	***Peptone medium***	Peptone + NaCl + water	For sugar fermentation test
B. Special **a. Enriched**	***1. Glucose broth***	Nutrient broth + glucose	For *Streptococcus*
	2. Hiss serum	Serum + peptone water	For *Corynebacterium*
b. Enrichment	***1. Selenite F broth***	Peptone water + sodium selenite	Isolation of *Salmonella* and *Shigella*
For specimens other than blood	***2. Tetrathionate broth***	Nutrient broth + sodium thiosulphate + calcium carbonate + iodine solution	For *Salmonella*
	3. Alkaline peptone water	Peptone water pH = 8.6	For *Vibrio cholerae*
Liquid media used for blood culture	***1. Brain heart infusion broth***	Nutrient broth + dehydrated heart meat	Blood culture
	2. Liver infusion broth	Nutrient broth + crushed lean liver of sheep	Blood culture of pyogenic bacteria and enteric bacilli
	3. Glucose broth	Nutrient broth + glucose	For pyogenic organism
	4. Bile broth	Nutrient broth + bile	For *Salmonella*

Biphasic media: Dispensed in blood culture bottles.

NAME OF MEDIUM	COMPOSITION	LABORATORY USE
Castaneda medium	***Brain heart infusion broth and agar***	For blood culture for Brucellosis

II. CULTIVATION OF ANAEROBIC BACTERIA

1. Culture Media (Anaerobic)

S. NO.	TYPE OF MEDIUM	NAME OF MEDIUM	COMPOSITION	LABORATORY USE
1.	**Liquid medium**	***Robertson Cooked medium***	**Nutrient broth + Minced meat**	**Growth of anaerobic bacteria**
2.	**Thioglycolate broth**	***Thioglycolate medium***	**Nutrient broth + 1% thioglycolate + Resazurin**	**Growth of anaerobic bacteria**

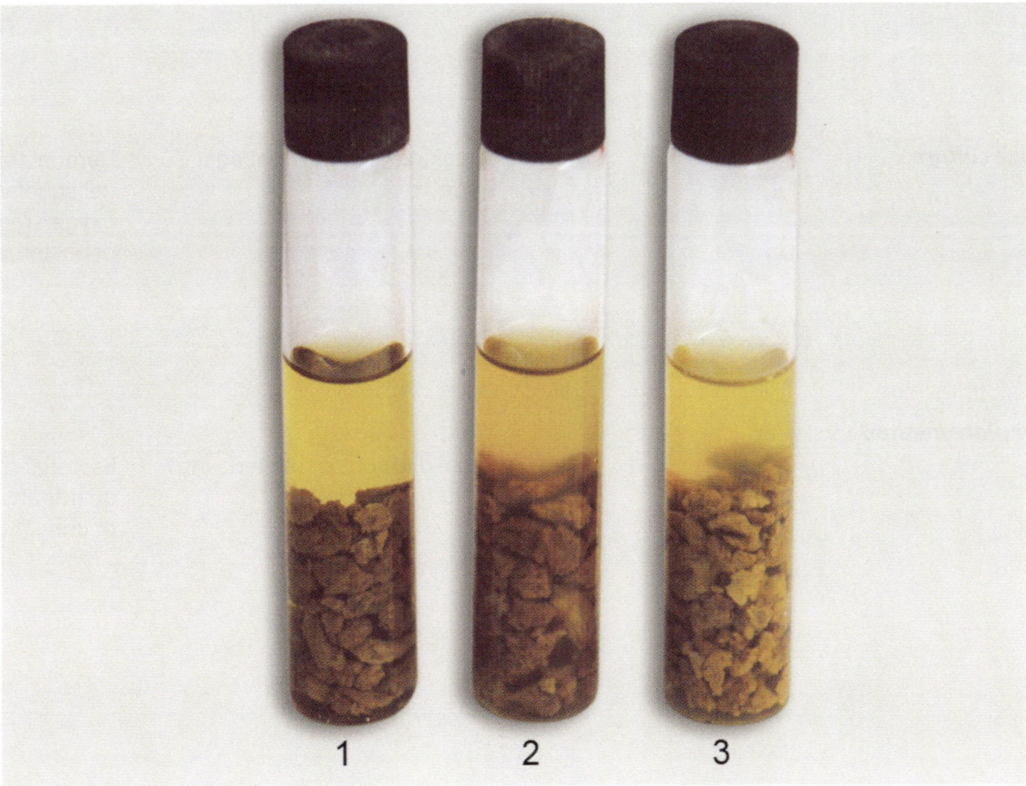

Cooked M Medium (RC medium) (M149)

1. Control
2. *Clostridium perfringens* ATCC 12924
3. *Clostridium sporogenes* ATCC 11437

Robertson Cooked medium

2. Inoculation Methods

Inoculation is done with a loop made of Nichrome wire of 24 S. W. G size; loop 2–4 mm. In diameter with a wire 2 to 3” long and is sterilized in the Bunsen flame. Various methods of inoculation are employed:

S. NO.	NAME OF METHOD	DIAGRAM	PROCEDURE	INDICATION
1.	***Streak culture***		Loop is sterilized on flame and inoculum is taken and smeared on a well From there create a parallel streaks A, B, C and the tail	To get isolated colonies
2.	***Lawn culture***		Hooding the plate with liquid culture suspension	For antibiotic sensitivity pattern
3.	***Stroke culture***		Streaking on a nutrient agar slope	Demonstration of gel liquefaction and oxygen requirements of bacteria
4.	***Pour plate method***		Serial dilutions of bacteria into molten agar	Bacterial count and quantitative analysis of urine

Q1. HOW ARE BACTERIA CATEGORISED ON THE BASIS OF THEIR OXYGEN AND TEMPERATURE REQUIREMENT?

On basis of their oxygen requirement

- **Obligate aerobes:** Those bacteria which require only oxygen for their growth, e.g. *Pseudomonas aeruginosa*
- **Facultative anaerobes:** Aerobes but can also grow without oxygen, e.g. *Staphylococcus* spp., *Escherichia coli*
- **Microaerophilic:** It can grow in presence of traces of oxygen, e.g. *Campylobacter jejuni, H. pylori*
- **Obligate anaerobes:** Obligate or strict anaerobes can grow only in the absence of oxygen, e.g. *Clostridium tetani*
- **Capnophilic:** Some bacteria require 5–10% amount of carbon dioxide for their growth, e.g. *Brucella abortus.*

On basis of their temperature

Mainly bacteria grow at 37°C. Bacteria are further grouped as:

- **Mesophiles:** Grows at temp. between 25°C and 40°C, e.g. all pathogenic bacteria
- **Psychrophiles:** Grows at temp. below 20°C, e g. Soil and water saprophytes
- **Thermophiles:** Grows at temp. between 55°C and 80°C, e.g. *Bacillus stearothermophilus.*

Incubator

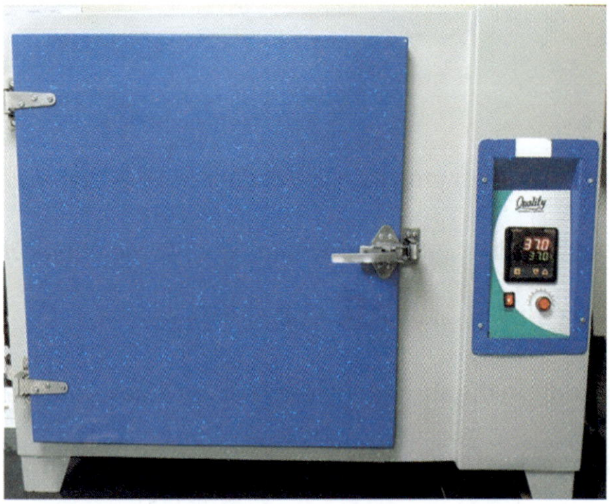	In microbiology, an incubator is a device used to grow and maintain microbiological cultures or cell cultures. The incubator maintains optimal temperature, humidity and other conditions. For routine bacterial cultures , temperature is maintained at 37°C.

McIntosh and Fildes' Anaerobic Jar

McIntosh and Fildes' anaerobic jar 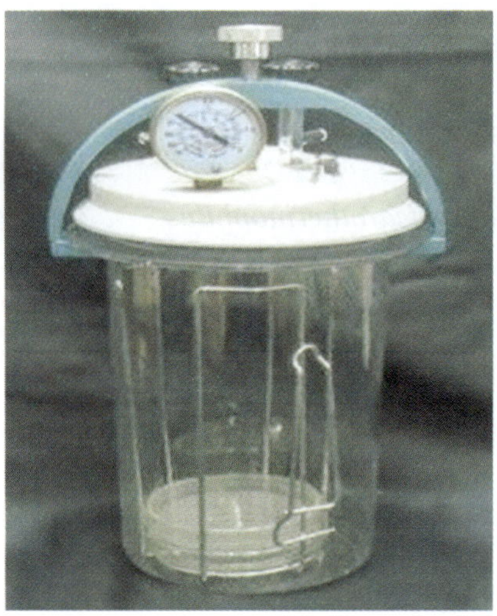	**McIntosh and Fildes' anaerobic jar** is an instrument used in the production of an anaerobic environment (anaerobiosis). Hydrogen gas is passed in Catalyst helps to combine hydrogen and oxygen. The presence of air is deleterious for many anaerobic bacteria and must be incubated in its absence. The inoculated culture plates are placed inside a metal jar and the lid clamped tight. The air inside is removed using a vacuum pump. The pressure inside the chamber is reduced to 100 mm below mercury.

Identification of Bacteria by Biochemical Reactions

8
CHAPTER

COMPETENCY

MI1.1: Describe the different causative agents of infectious diseases, methods used in their detection and discuss the role of microbes in health and disease.

1. CATALASE TEST

Principle: The enzyme catalase decomposes hydrogen peroxide (H_2O_2) into water and nascent oxygen. The presence of enzyme in a bacterial isolates is evident when a small inoculum is introduced into H_2O_2 and the rapid elaboration of oxygen bubbles occurs. The lack of catalase enzyme is evident by a lack of or weak bubble.

Procedure: With an inoculating needle or a wooden applicator stick, transfer growth from the centre of a colony to the surface of a glass slide. Add a drop of of 3% hydrogen peroxide and observe the bubble formation. This test is used to differentiate *Staphylococcus* spp. and *Streptococcus* spp.

Interpretation: The rapid and sustained production of bubbles or effervescence constitutes a positive test because of the production of enzyme catalase.

Quality control:

Positive control: *Staphylococcus aureus*

Negative control: *Streptococcus pyogenes.*

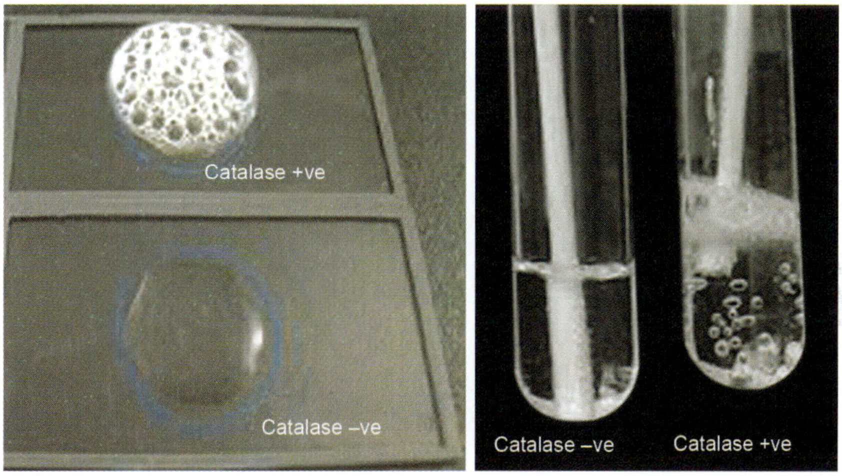

Catalase test

2. OXIDASE TEST

Principle: Cytochromes are iron-containing hemoproteins that act as the last link in the chain of aerobic respiration by transferring electrons (hydrogen) to oxygen, with formation of water. The cytochrome system is found in aerobic, microaerophilic and facultatively anaerobic organisms. The dye 1% solution of tetra methyl-para-phenylene-diamine dihydrochloride is oxidized to indophenol blue producing deep purple color.

Procedure: Wet filter paper method is used in this test. Strips of Whatman no.1 filter paper is soaked with a little freshly made 1% solution of tetra methyl-para-phenylene-diamine dihydrochloride and then with a help of sterile glass rod a single colony from the medium is rubbed over the strip.

Interpretation: A positive reaction is indicated by an intense deep purple blue color appearing within 5–10 seconds and a negative reaction by absence of coloration or by coloration later than 60 seconds.

Quality control:

Positive control: *Pseudomonas aeruginosa* ATCC 27583

Negative control: *Escherichia coli* ATCC 25922

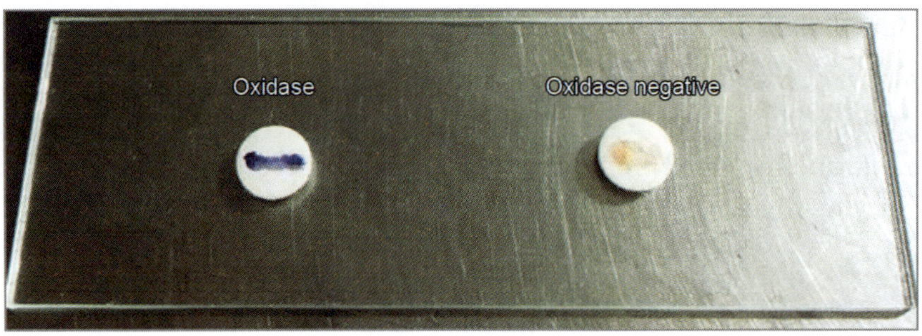

Oxidase test

3. COAGULASE TEST

This test is done to differentiate between Staphylococcus species. Both slide and tube coagulase test is done. Coagulase is present in two forms, bound and free, each having different properties that require the use of separate testing procedures.

Slide Coagulase Test

Principle: Slide coagulase test detects bound coagulase which is attached to the bacterial cell wall and is not present in culture filtrate. Fibrin strands are formed between the bacterial cells when suspended in plasma (fibrinogen), causing them to clump not visible aggregates.

Procedure: A smooth milky suspension of the growth is made in normal saline over a clean glass slide. Make similar suspension of control positive and negative strains to confirm the proper reactivity of the plasma. To the test suspension a loop full of undiluted human plasma is added and the suspension is observed for the appearance of coarse clumps.

Interpretation: It is read as positive when a coarse clumping of cocci is visible to the naked eye within 10 seconds. Negative is read when there is absence of clumping.

Tube Coagulase Test

Principle: Coagulase is a protein that has prothrombin-like activity which can convert fibrinogen to fibrin. A visible clot is seen. Heat labile protein secreted free into the medium and clots the rabbit plasma in presence of factor known as Coagulase Reactive Factor (CRF), which is similar to prothrombin present in plasma and converts fibrinogen into fibrin.

Free coagulase + CRF ⟶ CRF coagulase

Fibrinogen ⟶ Fibrin

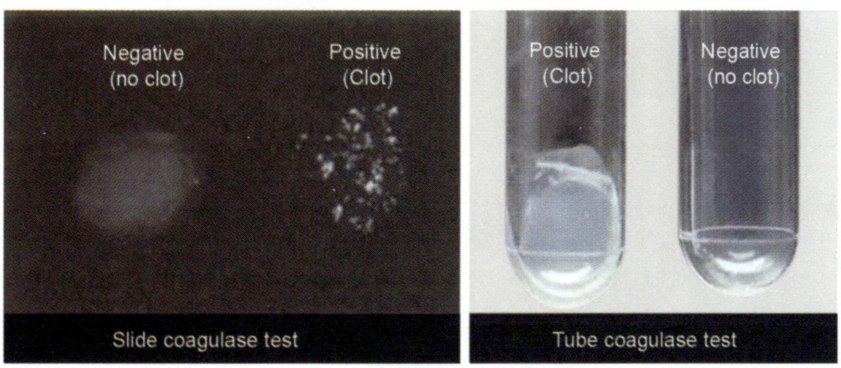

Coagulase test

4. INDOLE TEST

Principle: This test is done to demonstrate the ability of certain bacteria that possess enzyme tryptophanase, which are capable of hydrolyzing and demeaning tryptophan with the production of indole, pyruvic acid and ammonia. Indole, a benzyl pyrrole, is one of the metabolic degradation products of amino acid tryptophan.

Procedure: Kovac's reagent method is employed. Kovac's reagent preparation.

Amyl or isoamyl alcohol : 150 mL
p-dimethylaminobenzaldehyde : 10 g
Concentrated HCl : 50 mL

Individual colonies are inoculated on to peptone water and incubated at 37°C for 18–24 hours. To this 0.5 ml of Kovac's reagent is added and gently shaken.

Interpretation: Appearance of bright fuschia pink colored ring at the interface of reagent and the broth within seconds after adding the reagent is indicative of the presence of indole and is a positive test.

Quality control:
Positive control: *Escherichia coli* ATCC 25922
Negative control: *Klebsiella pneumonia.*

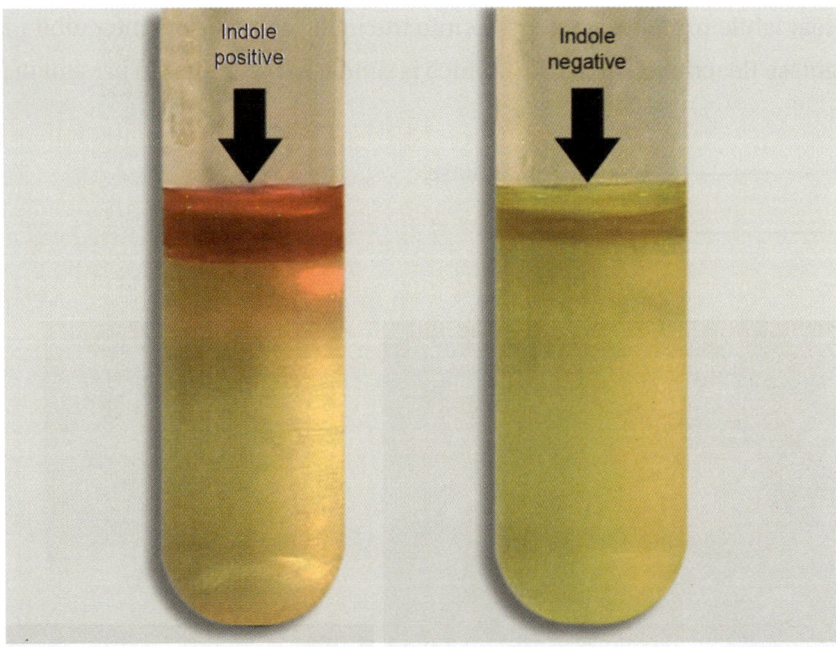

Indole test

5. UREASE TEST

Principle: Urease is an enzyme possessed by many species of microorganisms. This test is done to determine the ability of bacteria to decompose urea into ammonia. Christensen's urea agar medium is used. Indicator used is Phenol red.

Procedure: Inoculate heavily over the entire surface of Christensen's urea agar medium with the peptone water culture and incubate at 37°C. Examine after 4 hours and then overnight incubation.

Interpretation

Positive: When the indicator turned to pink-purple.

Negative: No change in color.

Quality control:

Positive control: *Proteus* species

Negative control: *Escherichia coli.*

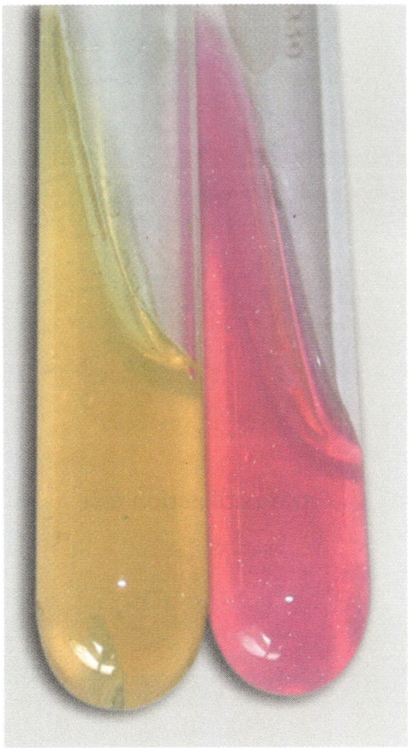

Urease test

6. CITRATE UTILIZATION TEST

Principle: The utilization of citrate by a test bacterium is detected in a citrate medium by the production of alkaline by products. To determine the ability of certain bacteria to obtain energy in a manner by utilizing citrate as a sole source of carbon for its growth. Simmon's citrate medium is used to know the utilization of citrate. Indicator is bromothymol blue.

Procedure: The citrate slant is inoculated with the suspected single colony and medium is incubated at 37°C for 24 to 48 hours. A positive reaction is indicated by the blue color and streak of growth. A negative reaction if original green color persists and no growth along the streak line.

Quality control:

Positive control: *Enterobacter aerogenes*

Negative control: *Escherichia coli.*

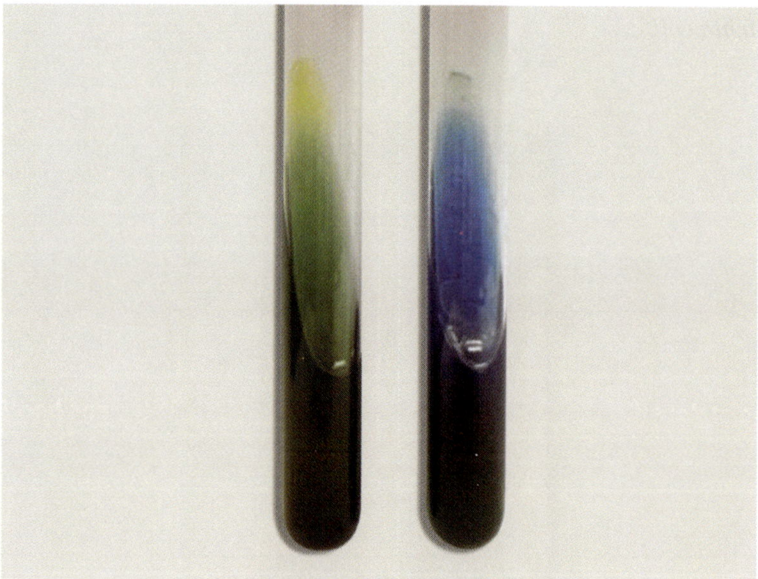

Citrate utilization test

7. TRIPLE SUGAR IRON AGAR TEST

Principle: This is done to determine ability of bacteria to ferment carbohydrates incorporated in a growth medium and production of hydrogen sulphide. Triple sugar iron (TSI) agar medium contains 10 parts Lactose, 10 parts Sucrose, 1 part glucose and peptone. Phenol red and ferrous sulphate serve as indicator of acidification and H_2S production respectively. With a sterile straight inoculating wire, touch the top of a well with isolated colony.

Procedure: Inoculate TSI slant by first stabbing through the center of the medium to the bottom of the tube and then streaking the surface of the agar slant. Incubate the tube at 37°C for 18–24 hours. The result is interpreted as follows:

Interpretation:

SLANT /BUTT	COLOR	UTILIZATION
Alkaline slant/acid butt (K/A)	Red/yellow	Glucose only fermented; peptone is utilized
Acid slant/acid butt (A/A)	Yellow/yellow	Glucose, lactose and/or sucrose fermented
Alkaline butt/alkaline butt (K/K)	Red/red	No fermentation of glucose, lactose or sucrose

A black precipitate in the butt indicates production of ferrous sulphide and H_2S gas. Bubbles or cracks in the media indicate the production of CO_2 or H_2.

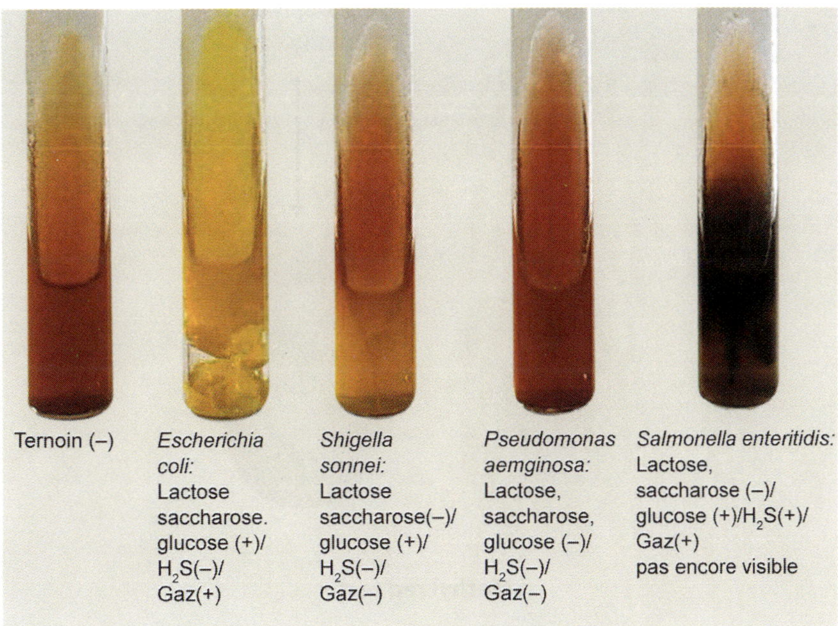

Triple sugar iron agar test

8. METHYL RED TEST

Principle: Methyl red is quantitative test for production of acid, requiring positive organism to produce string acids (lactic acid, acetic acid, formic acid) from glucose through the mixed acid fermentation pathway. This test is to determine the ability of bacteria which can maintain the low pH after prolonged incubation.

Procedure: Inoculate the glucose phosphate broth with a pure culture of test organism and incubate at 37°C for 48 hours (no fewer than 48 hours). To this, add about five drops of the methyl red reagent. Mix and read immediately.

Interpretation: Development of stable red color in the surface of the medium indicates sufficient acid production to lower the pH to 4.4 and constitutes a positive test.

Quality control:

Positive control: *Escherichia coli*

Negative control: *Enterobacter aerogenes.*

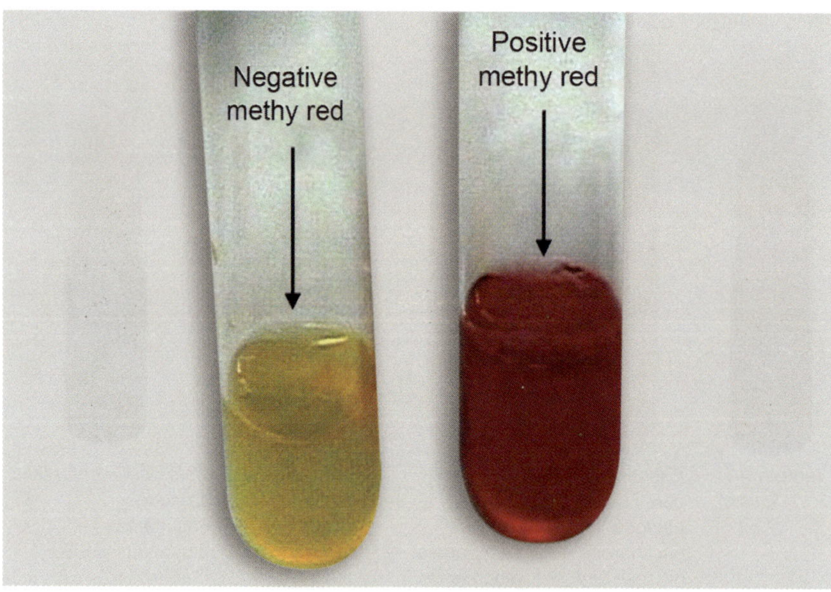

Methyl red test

9. VOGES PROSKAUER TEST

Principle: Pyruvic acid is a pivotal compound formed in the fermentative degradation of glucose, further metabolized through various metabolic pathways, depending upon the enzyme systems possessed by different bacteria, where the end product is acetoin (acetyl methyl carbinol). In the presence of atmospheric oxygen and 40% potassium hydroxide, acetoin is converted into diacetyl and alpha-naphthol serves as a catalyst to bring out a red complex.

Procedure: Inoculate the glucose phosphate peptone broth with a pure culture of test organism and incubate at 37°C for 48 hours. To this add 0.6 mL of 5% α-naphthol followed by 0.2 mL of 40% potassium hydroxide. Shake the tube gently to expose the medium to atmospheric oxygen and allow to remain it undisturbed for 10–15 minutes.

Interpretation: A positive reaction is indicated by the development of a red color in 15 minutes,indicating the presence of diacetyl, the oxidation product of acetoin. It turns crimson red in color in 30 minutes.

Quality control:

Positive control: *Enterbacter aerogenes*

Negative control: *Escherichia coli*

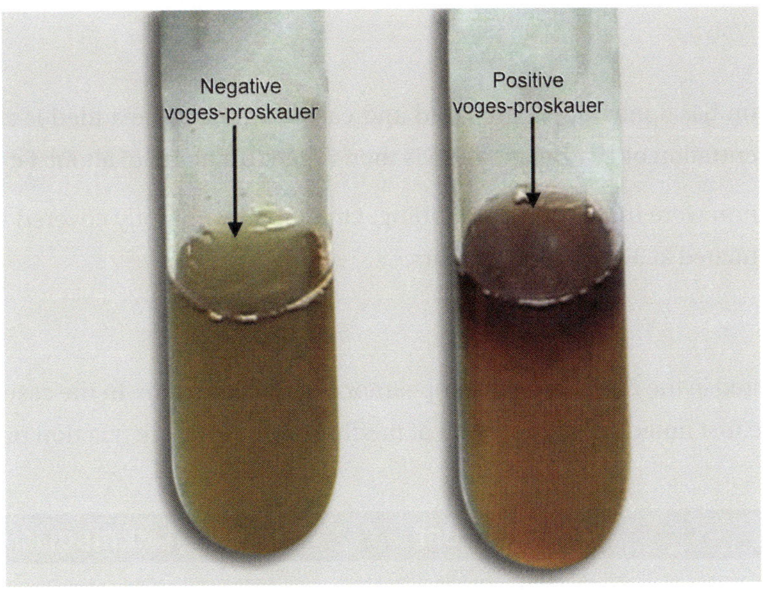

Voges-Proskauer test

10. SUGAR FERMENTATION TEST

Principle: This test is done to determine the ability of an organism to ferment a specific carbohydrate that is incorporated in a basal medium, thereby producing acid with or without visible gas.

Procedure: The test is performed on conventional culture media with test sugars. The common sugar fermentation media used are glucose, lactose, sucrose, maltose, mannose, arabinose and xylose. From the peptone water tube (which was incubated for 2 hours.after inoculation) all the sugar fermentation media are inoculated with the help of a Pasteur pipette. After the different media are inoculated, these are incubated at 37°C for 18–24 hours. After 24 hours the sugar media are examined for the production of acid indicated by pink color and gas (presence of an air bubble inside the Durham's tube).

Interpretation: Positive test is indicated by change in color to pink with or without gas formation in Durham's tube. Negative test is indicated by growth, but no change in color.

11. OXIDATION/FERMENTATION TEST (MODIFIED HUGH AND LEIFSON)

Principle: This test is done to know the organism uses carbohydrate substrate to produce acid by products either oxidatively or fermentatively.

Procedure: Hugh-Leifson basal medium is prepared and carbohydrate to be added is sterilized separately and added to give final concentration of 1%. The medium is then tubed to a depth of about 4 cm.

Duplicate tubes of medium were inoculated by stabbing. One tube is promptly covered with liquid paraffin to a depth of 1 cm and is incubated at 37°C for 18–24 hours.

Interpretation

Acid production is detected in the medium by the appearance of a yellow color. In the case of oxidative organisms, color production may be first noted near the surface of medium. Following are reaction patterns:

OPEN TUBE	COVERED TUBE	METABOLISM
Acid (yellow)	Alkaline (green)	Oxidative
Acid (yellow)	Acid (yellow)	Fermentative
Alkaline (green or blue)	Alkaline (green or blue)	Non-saccharolytic

12. NITRATE REDUCTION TEST

Principle: The test is used to determine the ability of an organism to reduce nitrate to nitrites which is used for the identification of family Enterobacteriaceae. The reduction of nitrate to nitrite is determined by adding sulfanilic acid and alpha-naphthylamine. The sulfanilic acid and nitrate forms a diazonium salt. The diazonium salt then couples with α-naphthylamine to produce a red, water soluble azo dye.

Procedure: This liquid medium is inoculated with the suspected single colony and the medium is incubated for 18–24 hours. Add 0.1 mL of the test reagent to the test culture. The test reagent is prepared by mixing equal volumes of solution A (8.0 g of sulfanilic acid in 1 L of acetic acid 5 mol/L) and solution B (5.0 g of α-naphthylamine in 1 L of acetic acid 5 mol/L).

Interpretation

Development of red color within 30 seconds after adding the test reagents indicates the presence of nitrites and represents a positive reaction for nitrate reduction.

Quality control

Positive control: *Escherichia coli*
Negative control: *Acinetobacter baumannii.*

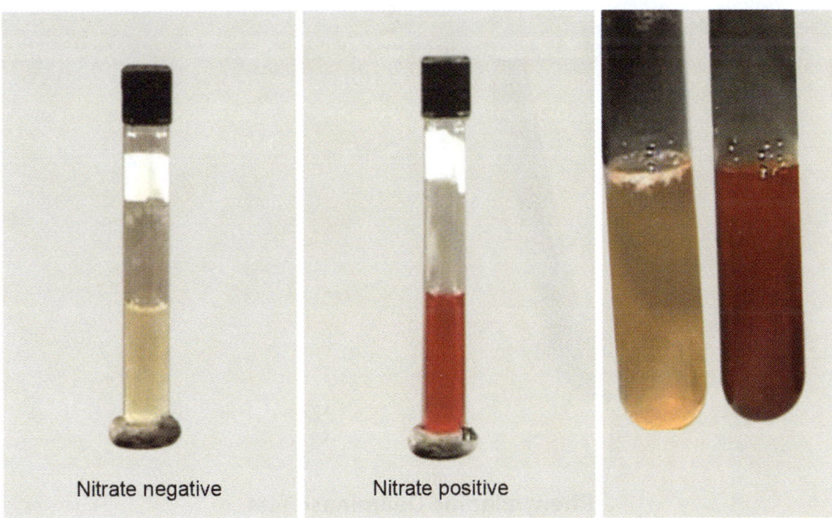

Nitrate reduction test

13. PHENYLALANINE DEAMINASE TEST (PPA)

Principle: To determine the ability of bacteria to deaminate phenylalanine to phenyl pyruvic acid (PPA). Of the enterobacteriaceae, only members of the *Proteus, Morganella and Providencia* genera possess the deaminase enzyme.

Procedure: This test was done to know the ability of the organism to deaminate phenylalanine with the production of phenyl pyruvic acid, which reacts with ferric salts to give green color. Inoculate it with pure growth and incubate 37°C for 18–24 hours. After incubation, allow a few drops of 10% solution of ferric chloride to run over the growth on the slope.

Interpretation: The immediate appearance of an intense green color indicates the presence of phenyl pyruvic acid and a positive test.

Quality control

Positive control: *Proteus* species

Negative control: *Escherichia coli.*

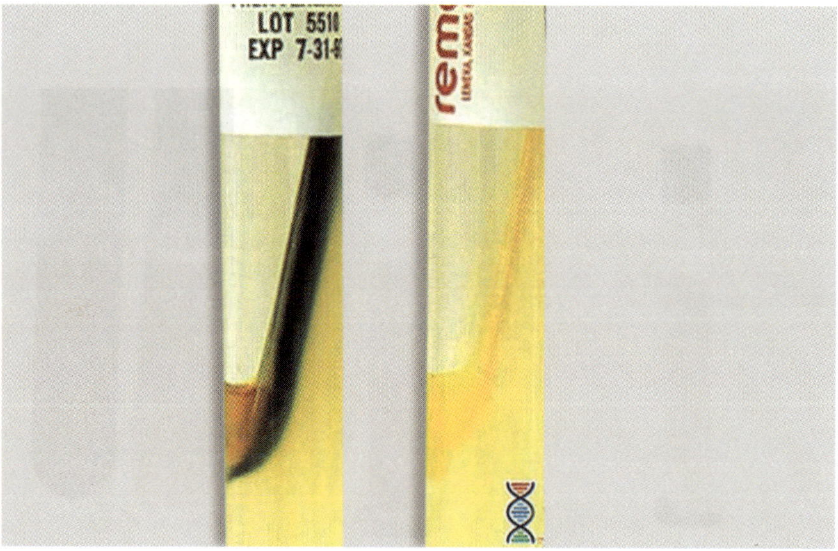

Phenylalanine Deaminase Test

14. AMINO ACID DECARBOXYLASES

Principle: Decarboxylases are group of substrate specific enzymes that are capable of reacting with the carboxyl portion of amino acids, forming alkalinel-reacting amines. The conversion of arginine to citrulline is a dehydrolase, in which an NH_2 group is removed from arginine. Citrulline is next converted to ornithine, which then undergoes decarboxylation to form putrescine.

Procedure: Two moller decarboxylases broth base is used. The amino acid to be tested is added to the decarboxylase base before inoculation with the test organism. A control tube, consisting only the base without the amino acid, must also be set up in parallel. Both tubes are anerobically incubated by overlaying the mineral oil. Incubate at 37°C for 18–24 hours. At initial stages of incubation, both the tubes turn yellow, owing to the fermentation of small amount of glucose in the medium. If amino acid is decarboxylated alkaline amines are formed and the medium reverts to original purple color. Indicators are cresol red and bromocresol purple.

L-lysine ——— lysine decarboxylase ———→ cadaverine + carbondioxide

Bromocresol purple ——— cadaverine ———→ bromocresol purple
(yellow) (lavender purple)

Interpretation

Conversion of the control tube to a yellow color indicates that the organism is viable and that the pH of the medium has been lowered sufficiently to activate the decarboxylase enzymes. Reversion of the tube containing the amino acid to a blue - purple color indicates a positive test owing to the formation of amines from the decarboxylation reaction.

Quality control

Amino acid	Positive control	Negative control
Lysine	*Enterobacter aerrogenes*	*Enterobacter cloacae*
Ornithine	*Enterobacter cloacae*	*Klebsiella pneumoniae*
Arginine	*Enterobacter cloacae*	*Enterobacter aerogenes*

Principles and Uses of Antimicrobial Agents

9
CHAPTER

COMPETENCY

MI1.6: Describe methods of antimicrobial susceptibility testing.

All strains of bacteria are not alike in their susceptibility to antimicrobial drugs. Therefore, the reliable guide to the therapeutic use of antimicrobial agents is an *In Vitro* sensitivity test. Two methods are generally in use.

1. DILUTION TEST

Serial dilutions of the drug in broth or agar are inoculated with the test organism and incubated overnight. The lowest concentration of the drug, i.e. the highest dilution in which the organism does not show growth is considered as the minimal inhibitory concentration (MIC) of the drug for the particular strain.

2. DISC DIFFUSION TEST

Six mm discs made out of Whatman filter paper are impregnated with antibiotics and preserved at 4°C in a refrigerator. The discs are impregnated with a standard quantity of the drugs. The medium used is Mueller-Hinton Agar on which a lawn culture is done and individual discs are placed. The plates are incubated overnight and inhibition of growth of the organism to each drug is estimated.

The Disc diffusion test can be done by two methods:

A. Stoke's Method

The zones of inhibition of the test organism are compared directly with those of the control stain of standard sensitivity, inoculated on the same plate.

B. Kirby Bauer's Method

The zones of inhibition of the test organism are compared with critical zone diameters given in a previously prepared scale. The scale correlates zone size with the MIC.

- The blood concentration achieved by the dose of anti-microbial prescribed, should be higher than MIC, but should not be toxic to the patient.

Practical 1

Record the drug sensitivity of the organism demonstrated, using Kirby Bauer's method.

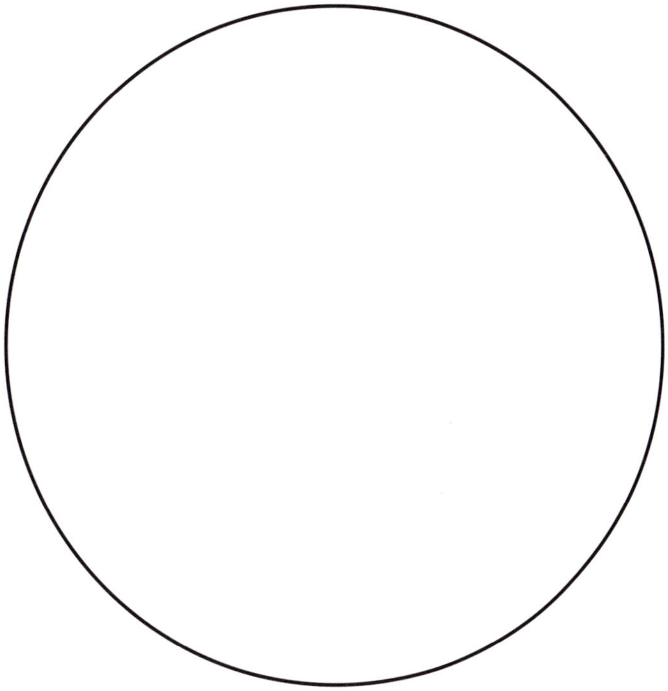

The given organism is:

Sensitive to:

Resistant to:

ANTIMICROBIAL STEWARDSHIP PROGRAM

COMPETENCY

PH 1.43: Describe the rational use of antimicrobials including antimicrobial stewardship program.

"**Antimicrobial stewardship**" refers to interventions designed to promote the optimal use of antibiotic agents, including drug choice, dosing, route, and duration of administration. To address antimicrobial resistance, all clinicians must become stewards of antimicrobials by prescribing them appropriately and educating their patients and colleagues on the proper use of this increasingly scarce medical resource.

Antimicrobial stewardship is a coordinated program that promotes the appropriate use of antimicrobials (including antibiotics), improves patient outcomes, reduces microbial resistance, and decreases the spread of infections caused by multidrug-resistant organisms.

Misuse and overuse of antimicrobials is one of the world's most pressing public health problems.

Infectious organisms adapt to the antimicrobials designed to kill them, making the drugs ineffective.

People infected with antimicrobial-resistant organisms are more likely to have longer, more expensive hospital stays, and may be more likely to die as a result of an infection.

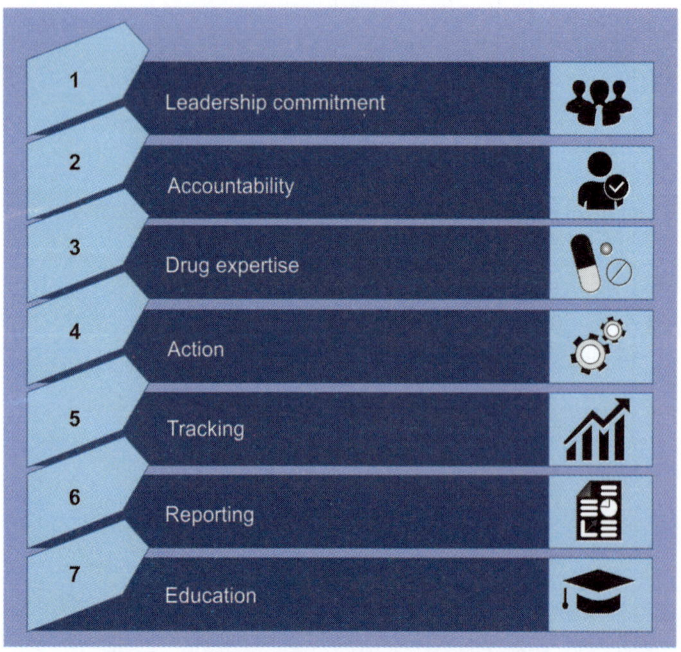

CDC's seven core elements of antimicrobial stewardship

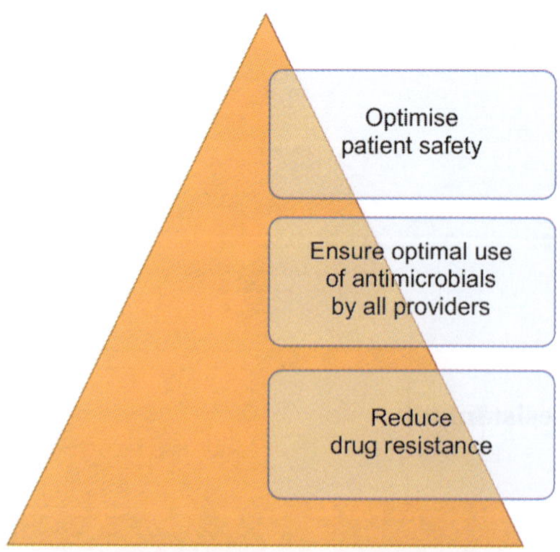

Goals of antimicrobial stewardship
***Source:* Department of Health (2013b)**

Section 2: Clinical Syndromes

Chapter 10: Collection and Transport of Clinical Specimens for Various Clinical Syndromes

Collection and Transport of Clinical Specimens for Various Clinical Syndromes

10
CHAPTER

COMPETENCY
MI8.9, MI8.10: Discuss the appropriate method of collection of samples in the performance of laboratory tests in detection of microbial agents causing infectious diseases.
MI8.11: Demonstrate respect for patient samples sent to the laboratory for performance of laboratory tests in the detection of microbial agents causing Infectious diseases.
MI8.14: Demonstrate confidentiality pertaining to patient identity in laboratory results.
MI8.15: Choose and interpret the results of the laboratory tests used in diagnosis of Infectious diseases.
PE 34.10: Discuss the various samples for demonstrating the organism in gastric aspirate, sputum, CSF, FNAC.

ETHICAL PROBLEMS IN LABORATORY EXAMINATIONS

Genetic testing, autopsy, prenatal and HIV examinations are ethically the most problematic laboratory examinations. The most problematic phase in the laboratory examination process proved to be the preanalytic phase. The most general problems of genetic examinations concerned maintaining confidentiality, protecting the autonomy of the subjects and questions of justice.

The basic principle of ethics dictates that individuals should be treated with respect and their dignity should not be violated. This respect must also extend to cover their culture values. Failure to respect the local cultural norms is regarded as the imposition of will and values of the dominant and powerful on the subordinate and marginal. The ethical problems in prenatal examinations mostly concentrated on **confidentiality**. **The ethical problems of HIV tests on autonomy and obtaining informed consent.**

Ethical Problems in the Preanalytic Phase

The main emphasis has been on ways to increase voluntary testing. General principles of professional conduct apply in the case of HIV testing. Relationships between health care providers and patients can be complex. These issues should be explored in the testing site's standard operational procedures and at each testing site director should make sure that all personnel are supported in developing their professional skills.

Informed consent for HIV testing means that the person being tested agrees to be tested on the basis of understanding the HIV testing procedures, the reasons for testing and is able to assess the personal implications. For some people with a heightened awareness of HIV, routine HIV testing may be a behavioral norm. For others with little understanding of HIV or their potential risk of exposure, HIV testing may be novel, frightening and perceived as highly stigmatising.

The person performing the test should use their professional judgement in securing informed consent. This should be based on their understanding of the context in which the test is being performed.

The features which precipitate testing such as clinical presentation, risk exposure, epidemiology and prevalence and patient initiation.

An assessment of the person being tested with respect to their understanding of the HIV testing process and consequences of the result.

Patients should also be advised how the test result will be conveyed.

Confidentiality

Confidentiality arises when there is a confidential relationship dependent on factors of trust, knowledge, and skill (e.g. doctor-patient relationships).

The patient has the right to confidentiality. The physician should not reveal confidential communications or information, without the consent of the patient, unless provided by law, for the need to protect the welfare of the individual, or for public interest. Civil and criminal penalties may ensue for unlawful disclosure of HIV positive status due to the negative connotations of a positive test for HIV (discrimination, psychological and social effects).

No healthcare provider, except a physician or a counsellor, shall disclose the HIV positive status of a person to his or her partner as per law, time to time.

1. BLOOD

COMPETENCY
IM1.22: Assist and demonstrate the proper technique in collecting specimen for blood culture.
IM3.10: Demonstrate the correct technique in a mannequin and interpret test results of a blood culture.
IM4.19: Assist in th e collection of blood and wound cultures.
IM25.9: Assist in the collection of blood and other specimen cultures.

Technique of Collection

- Select venipuncture site, then release tourniquet. Cleanse the selected venipuncture site.
- Rub vigorously with an alcohol prep pad. Let dry for 1 minute.
- Apply a 10% povidone-iodine solution over the same area, beginning at the proposed entry site and circling outward to a diameter of approximately 5 cm. Let dry for 1 minute.
- Cleanse the site a second time with an alcohol prep pad to remove the iodine by wiping down the center of the prep area, then down each side. This step is helpful in the event the site must be palpated during the phlebotomy procedure.
- Clean rubber caps of Vacutainer and blood culture containers with alcohol. Do not prep rubber stoppers with any other agent, per manufacturer's instructions.
- Retie tourniquet without touching the prepped area, insert needle into vein, and withdraw blood. After bleeding stops, if any iodine remains on the skin, reclean venipuncture site with alcohol to remove.
- Repeat the procedure for each blood culture set ordered, selecting a different site for each venipuncture, if possible.

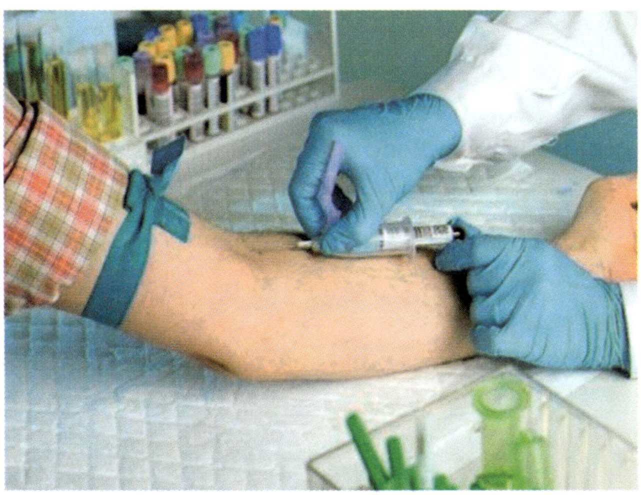

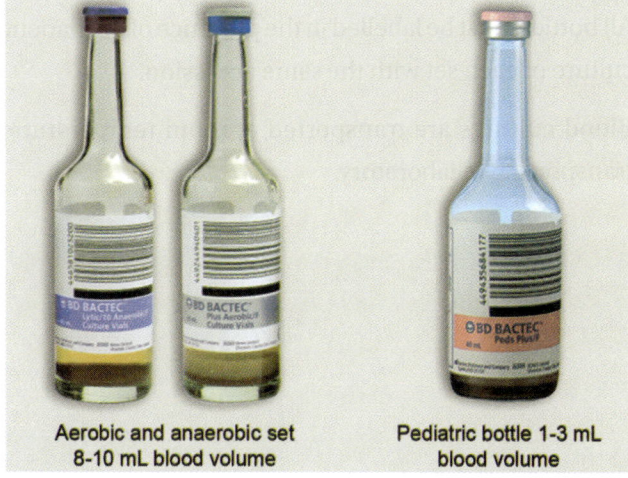

Aerobic and anaerobic set 8-10 mL blood volume

Pediatric bottle 1-3 mL blood volume

Tubes Commonly Used in Blood Collection and their Specifications

SAMPLE TYPE	TUBE TYPE	ADDITIVE	CAP COLOR
Blood culture (whole blood)	Blood culture bottle with variable content	None	Variable
Serum	No-additive tube (glass)	None	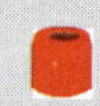
	Tube with clot activator	Clot activator	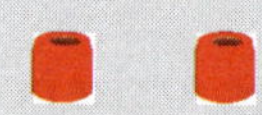
	Tube with gel/clot activator	Gel/clot activator	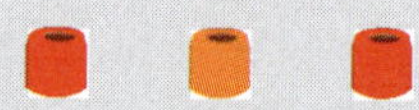
Plasma	Glucose tube	Sodium fluoride/potassium oxalate; Sodium fluoride/EDTA Sodium fluoride/Sodium heparin iodacetate/lithium heparin	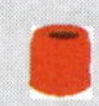
	Coagulation tube	Sodium citrate (9:1)	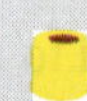
	Heparin tube	Sodium heparin lithium heparin	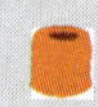
Whole blood	Tube with EDTA	EDTA K2 EDTA K3	
	ESR (sedimentation) tube	Sodium citrate (4:1)	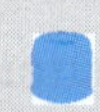

EDTA: Ethylenediamine tetraacetic acid; ESR: Erythrocyte sedimentation rate, (9:1), (4:1); blood/additive ratio

Labelling and Transport

All bottles must be labelled in the presence of the patient. Label the Vacutainers, aerobic/anaerobic bottles for blood culture of each set with the same accession.

Blood cultures are transported at room temperature. Do not refrigerate blood cultures, if there is a delay in transporting to laboratory.

DEFINE PUO ENUMERATE VARIOUS CAUSES OF PUO

Definition

Any febrile illness with a body temperature more than 38°C or more than 100°F, lasting for more than 3 weeks or longer, without any obvious cause or remain uncertain in spite of investigations.

Causes

Bacterial

LOCALIZED PYOGENIC INFECTIONS	SYSTEMIC BACTERIAL INFECTIONS
Appendicitis	Mycobacterial infections
Cholangitis	Typhoid fever
Cholecystitis	Mycoplasma
Localized abscess	Chlamydial infections
Mesentric lymphadenitis	Brucellosis
Osteomyelitis	Melioidosis
Pelvic inflammatory disease	Listeriosis
Sinusitis	Bartonellosis
Suppurative thrombophlebitis	Spirochetal infections
Intravascular infections	

Viral: Chikungunya fever, dengue fever, cytomegalovirus and EBV infection, Coxsackie group B, viral hepatitis, HIV infection.

Fungal: Aspergillosis, mucormycosis, blastomycosis, histoplasmosis, coccidioidomycosis, paracoccidioidomycosis, candidiasis, cryptococcosis, pneumocystis infection, sporotrichosis.

Parasitic: Malaria, amoebiasis, leishmaniasis, Chagas' disease, toxoplasmosis, strongyloidiasis.

LABORATORY DIAGNOSIS OF PYREXIA OF UNKNOWN ORIGIN

A. Microscopy

- **Blood microscopy:** Useful for detection of malarial parasites (ring and gametocytes), microfiariae, *Leishmania donovani* (LD forms or amastigote forms) and trypanosomes (trypomastigote form)
- **Stool wet mount:** For detection cyst, trophozoite or ova for *Entameoaba histolytica*
- **Gram stain:** of pus, sputum and other specimen can be carried out for detection of causative agent
- **Ziehl-Neelsen stain**: For *M. tuberculosis.*

B. Culture

- Blood culture is done for typhoid fever, brucellosis, septicemia, subacute bacterial endocarditis.
- Culture on Lowenstein-Jensen (LJ) media for *M. tuberculosis.*
- Culture for pus and exudates specimen to be inoculated on blood agar (BA), MacConkey agar (MA), chocolate agar (CA) for aerobic organism, Sabouraud dextrose agar (SDA) for fungal specimens and appropriate cell lines for isolation of virus for cytomegalovirus (CMV).

C. Serological Tests

- ELISA for rapid tests for viral infections like hepatitis, human immunodeficiency virus (HIV), cytomegalovirus (CMV), Epstein-Barr virus (EBV), dengue virus, chikungunya virus etc.
- Standard agglutination test: For brucellosis
- Microscopic agglutination test: For leptospirosis
- Cold agglutination test: For mycoplasma
- Weil-Felix test: For rickettsial diseases
- Paul- Bunnel test : For infectious mononucleosis
- Widal test: For enteric fever
- Microimmunofluorescence test or complement fixation test for chlamydial infections
- Rheumatoid arthritis (RA factor): For rheumatoid arthritis
- Antinuclear antibody detection by immunofluorescence or ELISA for diagnosis of systemic lupus erythematosus (SLE)
- Coagglutination test for *Salmonella typhi* antigen detection.

D. Molecular Test

Polymerase chain reaction (PCR).

E. Other Tests

- Complete blood count
- Raised ESR
- Imaging techniques.

CASE STUDY

MI 3.4: Identify the different modalities for diagnosis of Enteric fever. Choose the appropriate test related to the duration of illness.

Enteric fever is caused by *Salmonella typhi*, paratyphi A, B.

Sample collection: Blood sample in blood culture bottle is collected before administering antibiotics. Using sterile syringe, 5-10 mL blood is collected for adults.

Media used for subculturing blood:

- Nutrient agar: Translucent colonies
- Blood agar: Grayish white colored colonies
- MacConkey agar: Non-lactose fermenting colonies
- Wilson and Blair medium: Jet black colonies with metallic sheen.

Biochemical reactions: Catalase (+), oxidase (-), indole (-), methyl red (+), Voges-Proskauer (-), citrate (+), TSI–K/A with H_2S production at the junction of slant and butt. Glucose, maltose and mannitol are fermented.

Serological testing

Widal test is done by second week of fever.

Coagglutination test for antigen detection.

Other specimens collected for culture are: Stool, urine, fluid from roseolar rash, bone marrow, duodenal aspirates.

Test done: Widal tube agglutination test.

Timing of test is important, as antibodies begin to arise during end of first week. The titers increase during second, third and fourth week after which it gradually declines. The test may be negative in early part of first week.

Principle: Patients' suffering from enteric fever would possess antibodies in their sera which can react and agglutinate killed, colored Salmonella antigens in a tube agglutination test.

Requirements: Widal rack, round-bottomed Felix tubes, conical-bottomed Dreyer's tubes, water bath, doubly diluted patient serum in three-four rows, killed colored suspensions of S. typhi O antigen, S. typhi H antigen, S. paratyphi AH antigen and optionally S. paratyphi BH antigen.

Reading the results: The control tubes must be examined first, where they should give no agglutination.

- Agglutination of O antigen appears as a "matt" or "carpet" at the bottom. Agglutination of H antigens appears loose, wooly or cottony. The highest dilution of serum that produces a positive agglutination is taken as titer. The titers for all the antigens are noted.
- Baseline titer of the population must be known before attaching significance to the titers. The antibody levels of individuals in a population of a given area give the baseline titer.
- A titer of 100 or more for O antigen is considered significant and a titer in excess of 200 or more for H antigens is considered significant.
- Patients who have received vaccines against *Salmonella* may give false positive reactions. True untreated infection results in rise in titer whereas vaccinated individuals do not demonstrate any rise in titer.
- **Anamnestic response:** Those individuals, who had suffered from enteric fever in the past, sometimes develop anti-Salmonella antibodies during an unrelated or closely related infection. It can be differentiated from true infection by lack of any rise in titer on repetition after a week.

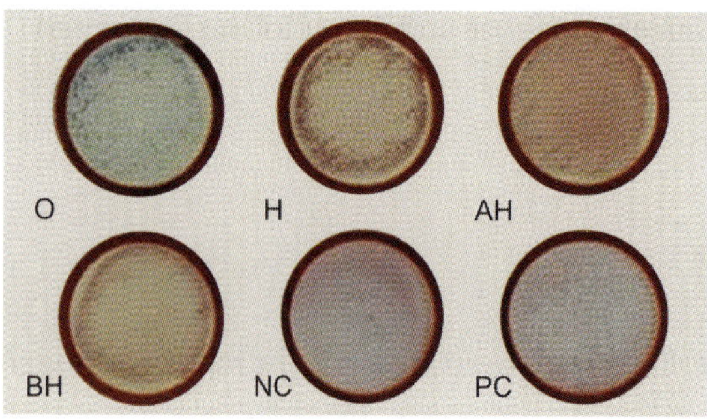

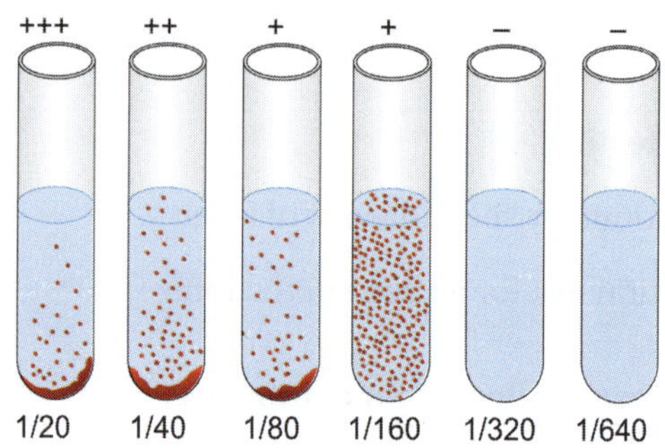

Widal test

2. CEREBROSPINAL FLUID

COMPETENCY

IM17.8: Demonstrate in a mannequin or equivalent the correct technique for performing a lumbar puncture.

Technique of Collection

- Identify interspaces and mark puncture site at the L4-5 interspaces in a perpendicular line from the iliac crest. Using sponge applicator provided in LP tray, prepare the back with Chlorhexadine solution, beginning at the site marked for the needle puncture and working outward.
- Repeat twice, drape the patient. Infiltrate the skin and subcutaneous tissue with preservative free 1% lidocaine with a 22-25-gauge needle.
- Insert the spinal needle into the midline of the interspaced with bevel up. Direct the needle on a 10-degree angle toward the umbilicus (horizontal axis).
- Advance the needle slowly, removing the stylet every 2-3 millimeters to check for CSF flow. Withdraw 2 millimeters, remove stylet and check for CSF. If none, then replace the stylet and remove. Remove the needle to subcutaneous tissue, change angle and continue.
- If repeated bony resistance is noted, discard the needle and replace it. If blood is returned, watch for clearing of fluid; if no clearing, replace the stylet.
- Once CSF flow is established, rotate the needle 90 degrees counter-clock wise (bevel in transverse plane) for patients in the lateral decubitus position. 1-2 mL of CSF in a universal container.
- Send samples to the lab for glucose, protein, cell count (culture and gram staining or other tests), cytology tests as indicated with proper labelling.

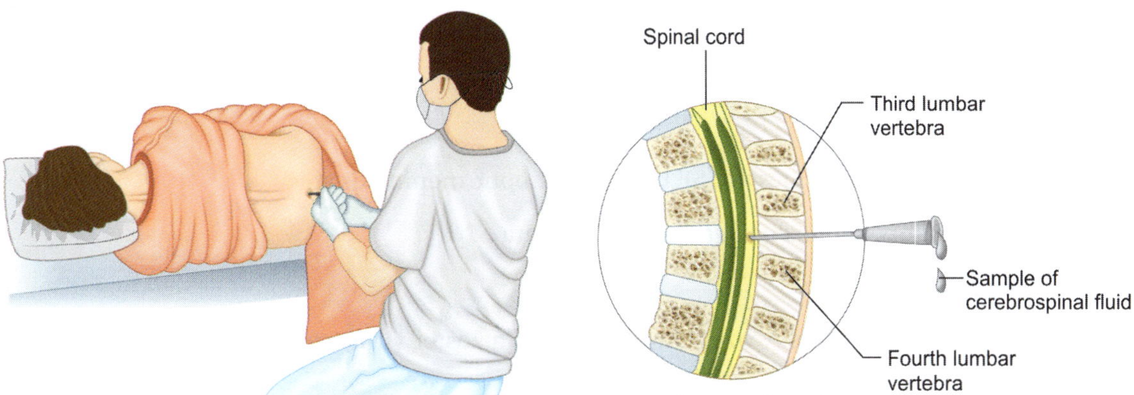

Position for lumbar puncture technique

Cross-section of blood the spine

Lumbar puncture

COMPETENCY
MI 5.3: Identify the microbial agents causing meningitis.
PA35.3: Identify the etiology of meningitis based on CSF parameters.
IM17.7: Enumerate the indications and describe the findings in CSF in patients with meningitis.
IM17.9: Interpret the CSF findings when presented with various parameters of CSF fluid analysis.
PE 30.21: Interpret and explain the findings in a CSF analysis.

Definition

Meningitis is an inflammation of the meninges surrounding the brain and spinal cord, which implies to infection of subarachnoid space or leptomeninges.

Types of Meningitis

Based on leukocytes in CSF, it is grouped into:

1. Pyogenic Meningitis

Characterized by elevated polymorphonuclear cells in CSF.

Causes of pyogenic meningitis are:

- Neonates or infants of 0–2 months–*Escherichia coli*, Group B *Streptococcus*, *Klebsiella pneumoniae*, *Listeria monocytogenes*
- 2-20 years: *Neisseria meningitidis, Haemophilus influenzae, Streptococcus pneumoniae*
- >20 years: *Streptococcus pneumoniae, Haemophilus influenzae* and *Neisseria meningitidis.*

2. Aseptic Meningitis

Characterised by elevated lymphocytes in CSF. Causes of aseptic meningitis are:

- **Bacteria:** *M. tuberculosis,Treponema pallidum*, Leptospira
- **Fungi:** *Cryptococcus neoformans*
- **Virus:** Enterovirus, herpes simplex virus 1 and 2, varicella zoster virus, cytomegalovirus, Epstein-Barr virus, mumps virus, arbovirus, adenovirus, rubella virus and HIV
- **Parasites:** *Naegleria fowleri, Acanthamoeba* spp., *Toxoplasma gondii.*

LABORATORY DIAGNOSIS OF COMMON ORGANISMS CAUSING MENINGITIS

AGENTS OF MENINGITIS	BIOCHEMICAL ANALYSIS	DIRECT DEMONSTRATION	CULTURE IDENTIFICATION
Streptococcus pneumoniae	Pyogenic meningitis CSF pressure TLC count: Highly elevated, neutrophilic (100-100000 per mm^3)	Gram positive cocci in pairs, lanceolate shaped	Alpha hemolytic, draughtsman shaped colony on blood agar, Sensitive to optochin, bile soluble, ferments inulin
Streptococcus agalactiae	Glucose- decreased to absent Total proteins: > 45 mg/dl (usually increased)	Gram positive cocci in short chains	Beta hemolytic pin point colony on blood agar Christie–Atkins–Munch-Peterson (CAMP) test positive Resistant to bacitracin
Neisseria meningitidis		Gram negative diplococci, intracellular, inside pus cells	Growth on chocolate agar, oxidase positive
Haemophilus influenzae		Pleomorphic gram negative bacilli	Satellitism on BA with *S. aureus* streak line, growth surrounding disc containing combined X and V factors
Escherichia coli and other gram negative organisms		Gram negative bacilli	Identification on MA and biochemical reactions
Cryptococcus neoformans	CSF pressure: Elevated or normal Leukocyte count: Slightly elevated and lymphocytic Glucose: Normal	India ink shows budding yeast cells with refractile capsule Latex agglutination test detecting capsular antigen in CSF	SDA, BA shows white mucoid colonies
Viral meningitis	Total proteins: Normal or slightly elevated	Detection of viral nucleic acid (DNA/RNA) by PCR	
Tubercular meningitis	CSF pressure: Moderately elevated, cobweb appearance Leukocyte count: Moderately elevated and lymphocytic Glucose: Slightly decreased Total proteins: Moderately to markedly increased	ZN stain of CSF shows acid fast bacilli Detection of specific genes in CSF by PCR or GeneXpert	Growth on LJ medium, rough, tough, buff colonies Growth on MGIT

3. SPUTUM

COMPETENCY

MI6.3: Identify the common etiologic agents of lower respiratory tract infections.

Technique of Collection

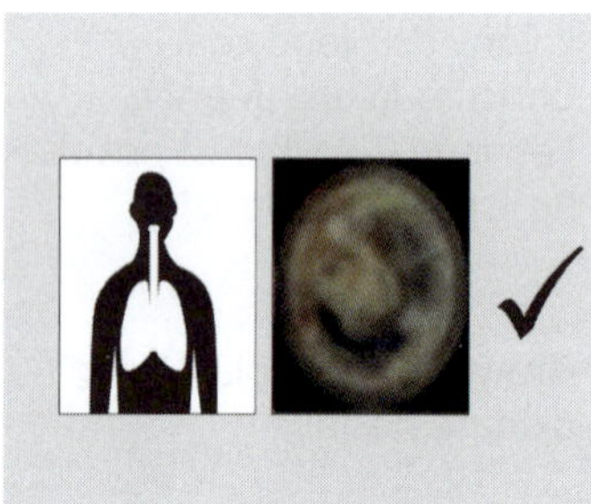

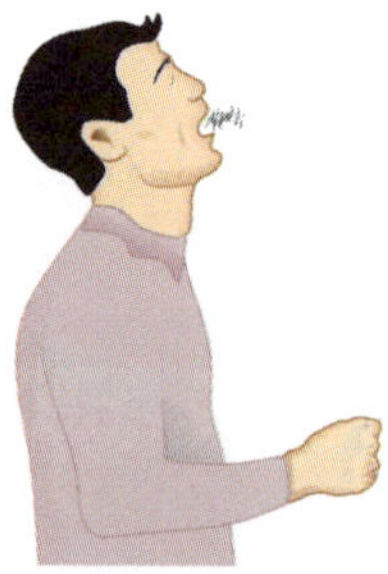

1. Gargle of rinse and then spit out the water you are given

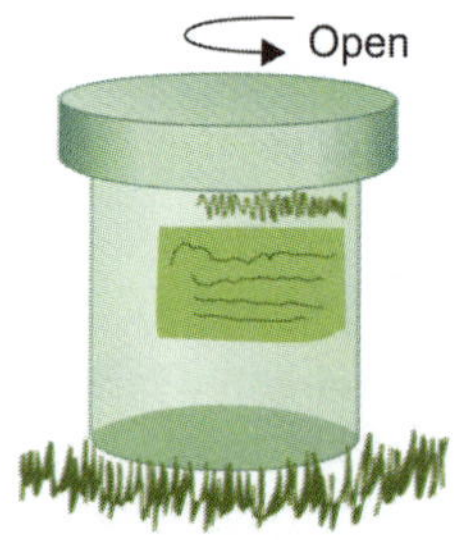

2. Open the sample container

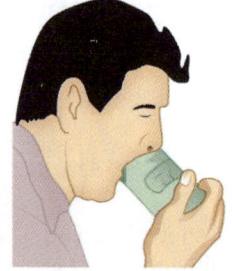

3. Hold the container to your mouth with your lips inside it

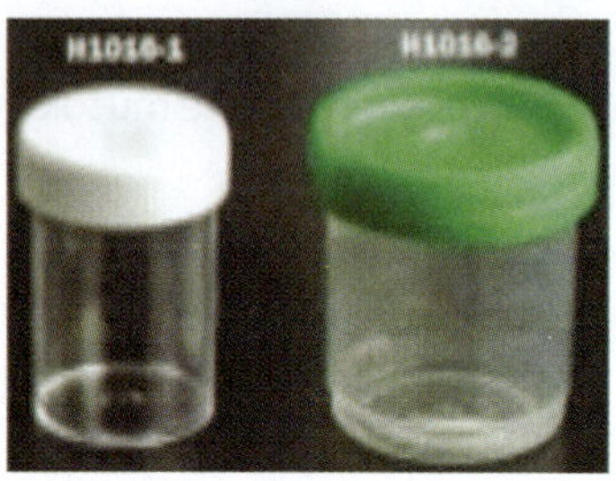

4. Take as deep a breath as you can and cough then spit into the container (do not just spit saliva)

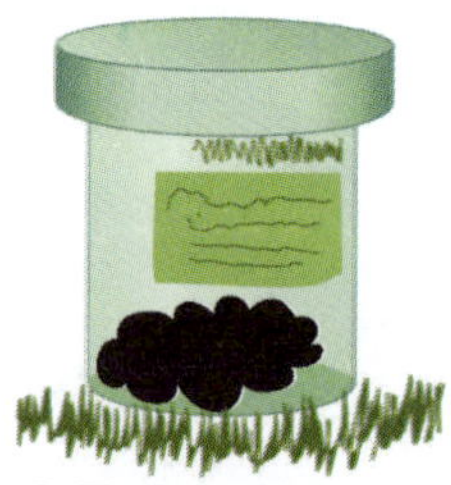

5. The sample you cough should look thick and yellow or green, more than a tablespoon of sample is needed

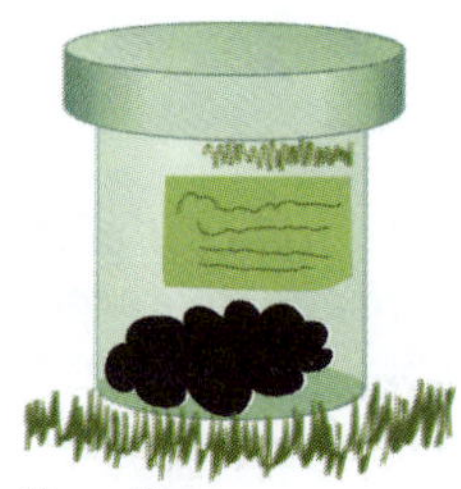

6. Close the container lid tightly and seal with parafilm

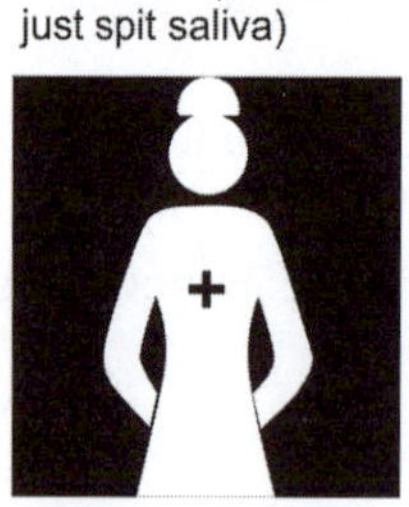

7. Give the sample to your caregiver right away

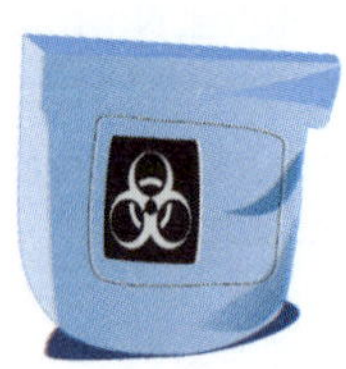

8. If you are at home
   - Put your sample in the plastic bag you were given
   - Close the bag and put it in the fridge right away
   - Return your sample to your caregiver within 24 hours

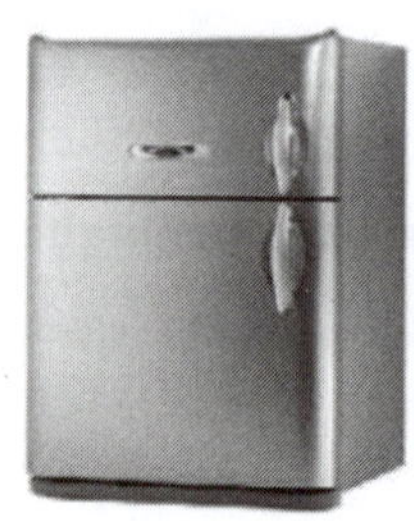

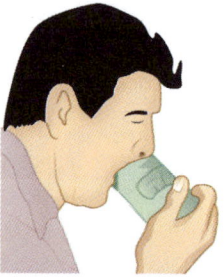

MENTION THE VARIOUS ORGANISMS CAUSING PNEUMONIA OR LOWER RESPIRATORY TRACT INFECTIONS AND ITS LABORATORY DIAGNOSIS.

Definition

Pneumonia refers to inflammation of lungs which can be classified as:

- ***Community acquired:*** Patients acquire organisms from community.
  - **Bacterial causes:** *Streptococcus pneumoniae, Mycoplasma pneumoniae, Haemophilus influenzae, Chlamydophila pneumoniae, Leigonella, Coxiella burnetii* (Q fever)
  - **Viral causes:** Influenza virus, adenovirus, respiratory syncytial virus, parainfluenza virus
- ***Hospital acquired:*** Patients acquire organisms in hospital setting
  - **Bacterial causes:** MDR Non-fermenters (*Pseudomonas* and *Acinetobacter* spp.), MDR Enterbacteriaceae (*E. coli, Klebsiella, Enterobacter), Streptococcus pneumoniae, Mycoplasma pneumoniae, Haemophilus influenzae, Chlamydophila pneumoniae, Legionella pneumoniae, Staphylococus aureus*
  - **Viral causes:** Influenza virus, adenovirus, respiratory syncytial virus, parainfluenza virus.

LABORATORY DIAGNOSIS FOR COMMON ORGANISMS CAUSING PNEUMONIA

Lobar Pneumonia

AGENTS OF PNEUMONIA	DIRECT DEMONSTRATION IN SPUTUM	CULTURE IDENTIFICATION
Streptococcus pneumoniae	Pus cells >25/LPF and epithelial cells <5/LPF Gram-positive cocci in pair, lanceolate shaped	Alpha hemolytic , draughtsman shaped colonies on blood agar, sensitive to optochin, bile soluble, ferment inulin
Haemophilus influenzae	Pus cells >25/LPF and epithelial cells <5/LPF, Pleomorphic gram-negative bacilli	Satellitism on blood agar with *Staph. aureus* streak
Staphylococcus aureus	Pus cells >25/LPF and epithelial cells <5/LPF, gram-positive cocci in clusters	NA- golden yellow colonies BA- beta haemolytic colonies Catalase positive, Coagulase positive
Gram negative bacilli (E. coli, Klebsiella, Pseudomonas, etc.)	Pus cells >25/LPF and epithelial cells <5/LPF, gram-negative bacilli	On MA (LF/NLF colony) Biochemical reactions

Interstitial or Atypical Pneumonia

AGENTS OF PNEUMONIA	DIRECT DEMONSTRATION IN SPUTUM	CULTURE IDENTIFICATION
Chamydophila pneumoniae	Direct Immunofluorescence test Antigen detection by enzyme immunoassay Nucleic acid amplification test(NAAT)	Serology-antibody detection by CFT using LPS antigen ELISA using recombinant LPS antigen Micro-IF test using outer membrane protein antigen
Mycoplasma pneumoniae	Direct Immunofluorescence test	Culture- fried egg colonies on PPLO agar Cold agglutination test ELISA
Legionella pneumoniae	Pus cells >25/LPF and epithelial cells <5/LPF. Detection of specific antigen in sputum, urine	Growth on BCYE agar
Viral pneumonia	Detection of specific viral antigen in sputum, detection of viral genes by PCR	

4. SORE THROAT

COMPETENCY
MI2.3: Identify the microbial agents causing Rheumatic Heart Disease and Infective Endocarditis.
MI6.2: Identify the common etiologic organisms of upper respiratory tract infections.

Technique of Collection

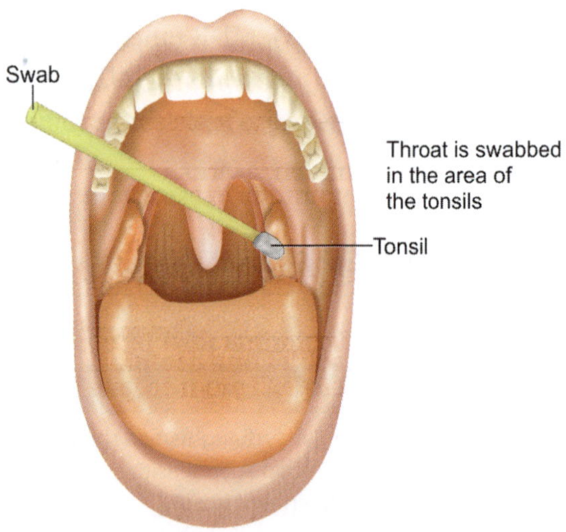

Throat swab

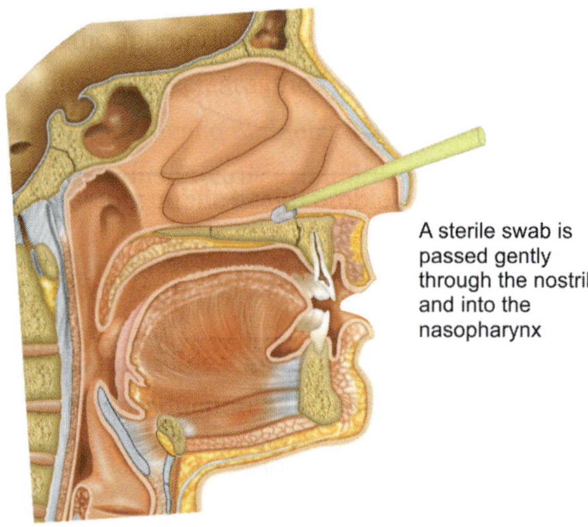

Nasopharyngeal swab

Mention the Various Organisms Causing Sore Throat

- **Bacterial:** *Streptococcus pyogenes* (most common), *Streptococcus pneumoniae, Corynebacterium diphtheria, Corynebacterium ulcerans, Treponema vincentii, Leptotrichia buccalis, Arcanobacterium* spp.
- **Fungal:** *Candida albicans*
- **Viral:** Influenza virus, parainfluenza virus, coxsackie virus, rhinovirus, coronavirus (MeRS Cov, NCOVID-19), Epstein-Barr virus, adenovirus.

5. URINE

COMPETENCY

MI7.3: Describe etiology, appropriate method of specimen collection for diagnosis of UTI.

Technique of Collection

In a universal container urine should be collected.

- **Clean voided midstream urine:** Most common specimen for UTI, collected after properly cleaning the urethral meatus or glans.
- **Suprapubic aspiration:** Urine from bladder, most ideal specimen. Recommended for infants or patients in coma.
- **In catheterized patients,** urine is collected from catheter tube (after clamping and disinfecting); but not from urobag.
- **Transportation of urine sample** should be done immediately. If delay, it can be refrigerated and stored by adding boric acid.

What are the various causative agents of urinary tract infection? What is Kass criteria?

Definition: Urinary tract infection is defined as disease caused by microbial invasion of the urinary tract that extends from renal cortex of kidney to urethral meatus.

UTI is classified into two types:

1. ***Upper UTI:*** Involves kidney and ureter.
2. ***Lower UTI:*** Involves urethra and bladder.

Bacteria:

- Gram negative: *Escherichia coli, Klebsiella pneumoniae, Proteus mirabilis, Pseudomonas aeruginosa, Acinetobacter* spp., *Enterobacter* spp., *Serratia* spp.
- Gram positive cocci: *Staphylococcus saprophyticus, Staphylococcus aureus, Staphylococcus epidermidis, Enterococcus* spp.

Viral: Herpes simplex virus, adenovirus, JC and BK virus, cytomegalovirus

Fungal: *Candida albicans*

Parasitic: *Schistosoma haematobium, Trichomonas vaginalis.*

Kass Criteria (Significant Bacteriuria):

Presence of bacteria more than 10^5 CFU/mL in a midstream urine sample by standard loop technique on Blood agar/Cystine-lactose-electrolyte-deficient (CLED) agar. It indicates active infection.

LABORATORY DIAGNOSIS OF COMMON ORGANISMS CAUSING UTI

Direct examination: Wet mount examination to demonstrate pus cells in urine.

- Leukocyte esterase test—to detect the esterase enzyme liberated by leukocytes
- Nitrate reduction test (Greiss test)—to detect nitrate reducing bacteria
- Catalase test—to detect catalase producing bacteria.

ORGANISMS	CULTURE	CULTURE SMEAR AND MOTILITY	BIOCHEMICAL REACTIONS
Escherichia coli	MA/CLED- flat, lactose fermenting colonies BA-gray moist colonies	GNB, motile	Catalase (+), Oxidase (-), Indole (+), MR (+), VP (-), Citrate (-), TSI (A/A) with gas
Klebsiella pneumoniae	MA/CLED- mucoid lactose fermenting colonies BA- gray mucoid colonies	GNB, non-motile	Catalase (+), Oxidase (-), Indole (-), MR (-), VP (+), Citrate (+), TSI (A/A) with abundant gas
Proteus spp.	MA/CLED- non-lactose fermenting colonies BA- swarming seen	Gram-negative pleomorphic bacilli, motile	Catalase (+), Oxidase (-), Indole (-/+), MR (+), VP (-), Citrate (-/+), Urease (+) TSI (K/A) with H2S PPA (+)
Staphylococcus aureus	NA- golden yellow colonies BA- beta hemolytic colonies	Gram-positive cocci arranged in clusters and short chains, non-motile	Catalase (+), Coagulase (+)
Staphylococcus saprophyticus	BA- white, non-hemolytic colonies	Gram-positive cocci arranged in clusters, non-motile	Catalase (+), Coagulase (-), Resistant to novobiocin
Enterococcus spp.	BA- translucent non-hemolytic colonies, MA- pink colonies	Gram-positive cocci arranged in pairs, spectacle shaped, non-motile	Catalase (-), Bile esculin (+)

CASE STUDY

A 30-year-old female comes to the outpatient department complaining of burning micturition and fever with chills and rigor. A midstream urine sample collected aseptically is subjected to culture and biochemical reactions were illustrated.

Causative organism: *Escherichia coli* causing UTI

Culture media: Blood agar, MacConkey's agar, CLED agar

Grams and motility: Gram negative bacilli, actively motile

Biochemical reactions of *E. coli:*

Catalase (+), oxidase (-), indole (+), methyl red (+), Voges-Proskauer (-), citrate (-), urease (-)

Triple sugar iron (TSI): Ferments glucose, lactose and sucrose with acid gas production (A/A with or without gas)

Also ferments maltose, mannitol.

Significant Bacteriuria: Kass Criteria

Presence of bacteria more than 10^5 CFU/mL in a midstream urine sample by standard loop technique on Blood agar/CLED agar. It indicates active/ acute infection.

- Colony count between 10^4 to 10^5 CFU/mL indicates doubtful significance, should be clinically correlated.
- Low count of $<=10^4$ CFU/mL is insignificant, indicates the presence of commensal bacteria.
- Quantitative culture such as pour plate method is carried out to count the number of colonies.

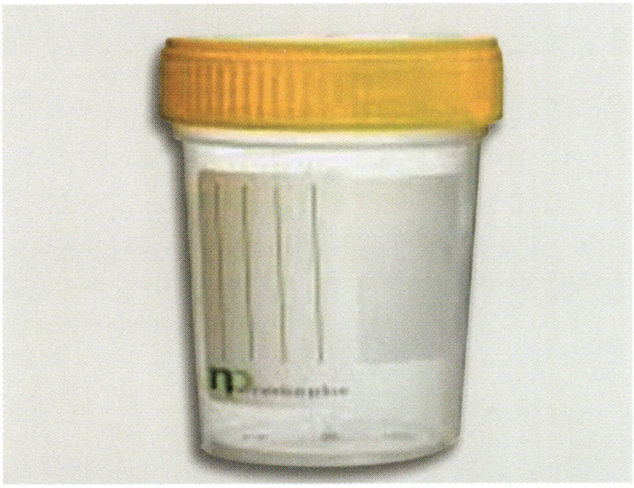

Universal container for collection of urine sample

6. VAGINAL SWAB/URETHRAL SWAB

COMPETENCY
MI7.2: Describe etiology, discuss laboratory diagnosis of sexually transmitted diseases. Recommend preventive measures.
DR10.7: Identify and differentiate based on clinical features of non-syphilitic sexually transmitted diseases (Chancroid, donovanosis, LGV).

Technique of Collection

High vaginal swab: For cervicitis, vaginitis

Urethral smear/exudates: Syphilis, chancroid, gonorrhoea, non-gonococcal urethritis.

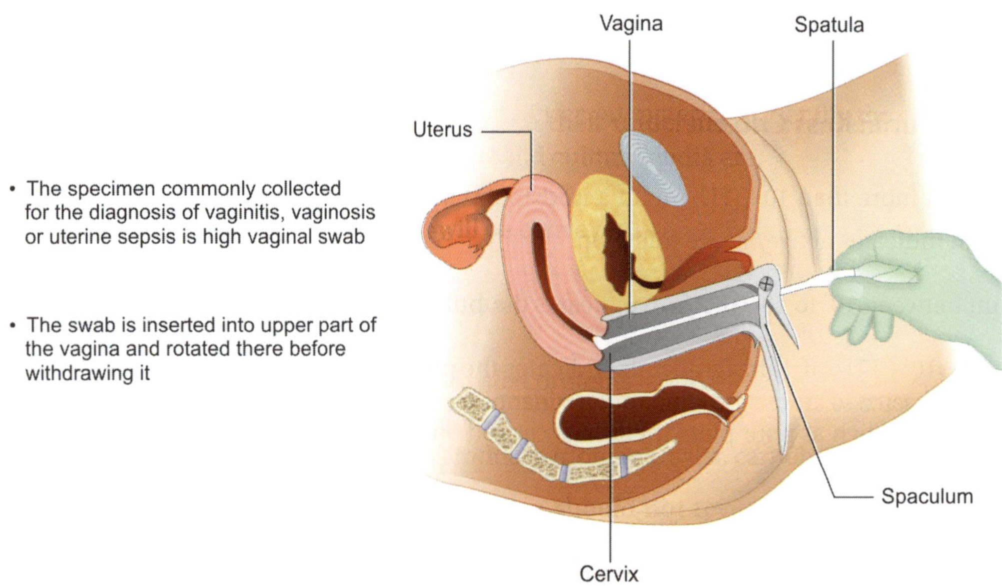

• The specimen commonly collected for the diagnosis of vaginitis, vaginosis or uterine sepsis is high vaginal swab
• The swab is inserted into upper part of the vagina and rotated there before withdrawing it
Vagina
Spatula
Uterus
Spaculum
Cervix

Collection of specimens

MENTION THE VARIOUS ORGANISMS CAUSING SEXUALLY TRANSMITTED DISEASES AND ITS LABORATORY DIAGNOSIS.

Definition: STDs are group of communicable diseases which are transmitted predominantly or entirely by sexual contact and caused by bacteria, virus, protozoa and fungus.

Classification Based on Clinical Manifestations

Painless Genital Ulcer

- Syphlis: *Treponema pallidum*
- Lymphogranuloma venereum: *Chlamydia trachomatis*
- Donovanosis: *Klebsiella granulomatis.*

Painful Genital Ulcer

- Chancroid: *Haemophilus ducreyi*
- Herpes genitalis: HSV1 and 2.

Urethral Discharge

- Gonorrhea: *Neisseria gonorrhoeae*
- Nongonococcal urethritis: *Chlamydia trachomatis, Ureaplasma urealyticum, Mycoplams genitalis, Mycoplasma hominis*, Herpes Simplex virus, *Candida albicans, Trichomonas vaginalis.*

Vaginal Discharge

- Vulvovaginal candidiasis: *Candida albicans*, non-albicans *candida*
- Bacterial vaginosis: *Gardnerella vaginalis, Mobiluncus* spp.
- Trichomonas vaginitis: *Trichomonas vaginalis.*

Genital Wart

Human papilloma virus.

Systemic Manifestations

Pelvic inflammatory disease: *N. gonorrhoeae* and *C. trachomatis*

No genital lesions: HIV, HBV, HCV.

LABORATORY DIAGNOSIS OF SEXUALLY TRANSMITTED DISEASES

Microscopy

- **Wet mount** for vaginal discharge:
  - In Trichomoniasis: Pus cells along with motile trophozoites are seen
  - In Candidiasis: Yeast cells along with pseudohyphae are seen
- **Gram-stained smear** of discharge or swab:
  - Bacterial vaginosis (*Gardnerella vaginalis*): Clue cells are seen, vaginal epithelial cells with gram-variable coccobacilli
  - Gonorrhea: Intracellular kidney shaped, gram-negative diplococci are seen
  - Candidiasis: Gram-positive budding yeast cells along with pseudohyphae are seen
- **Giemsa Stain:**
  - *Klebsiella granulomatis*: Presence of Donovan bodies (macrophage filled with bipolar stained bacilli)
  - *Chlamydia trachomatis*: Inclusion bodies
- **Dark ground microscopy and Silver impregnation method** in Syphilis: Spiral shaped coiled bacilli with corkscrew motility.

Culture

- Thayer Martin medium: *N. gonorrhoeae*
- Chocolate agar added with Isovitalex and Vancomycin: *Haemophilus ducreyi*
- McCoy cell line: *Chlamydia trachomatis*
- Sabouraud's dextrose agar: *Candida albicans*
- Cell lines such as Vero cells, monkey kidney cell line for Herpes simplex virus.

Serology

- Non-specific tests for syphilis: VDRL (venereal disease research laboratory) or RPR (rapid plasma reagin)
- Specific tests: TPHA, TPA, FTA-Abs.

Molecular Test

Multiplex PCR and Real-time PCR for *C. trachomatis, N. gonorrhoeae, T. pallidum, H. ducreyi* and HSV.

7. PUS SAMPLE

COMPETENCY
MI4.1: Enumerate the microbial agents causing anaerobic infections. Describe laboratory diagnosis of anaerobic infections.
MI4.3: Describe etiopathogenesis of infections of skin and soft tissue and its laboratory diagnosis.

Technique of Collection

For Aerobes

- Samples of pus are preferred in swabs. However, pus swabs are often received (when using swabs, the deepest part of the wound should be sampled, avoiding the superficial microflora). Swabs should be well soaked in pus. Swabs for bacterial and fungal culture should be placed in the transport medium provided in the tube.
- If possible a few mL of pus in a sterile universal bottle or even a few drops still in a syringe is much better than a swab. (The syringe must be safely capped and needles should NOT be sent).
- Ideally, a minimum volume of 1 mL of pus.
- Two wound swabs were collected from the wound and from a drop of aspirate, smear was made on clean glass slide and Gram staining was done for direct microscopic examination under oil immersion 100X objective to know various morphological types of bacteria and presence or absence of inflammatory cells.
- Second swab/drop of aspirate was used for culture by inoculating it on routine media like Blood Agar, Nutrient Agar and MacConkey's Agar, incubated at 37°C for 24 hours aerobically.

For Anaerobes

Ideally, a minimum volume of 1 mL (up to 5 mL) of pus should be collected. Large volumes of purulent material maintain the viability of anaerobes for longer. The aspirate should be collected in a sterile syringe - any air bubbles should be expelled. Syringe safely and tightly capped.

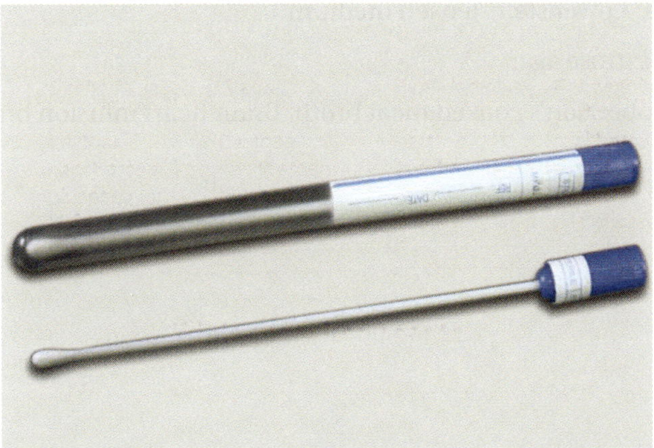

Etiology of Infections of Subcutaneous Tissue

- **Bacteria:** *Clostridium perfringens, Clostridium novyi, Clostridium septicum, Bacillus* spp., *Bacteroides* spp., *Peptostreptococcus* spp., *Staphylococcus aureus*, Group A *Streptococcus*
- **Fungi:** *Madurella mycetomatis, Madurella grisea, Candida* spp.
- **Parasites:** *Taenia solium, Wuchereria bancrofti, Dracunculus medinensis.*

Agents Causing Surgical Site Wound Infections

- **Bacterial**: *Staphylococcus aureus*, Coagulase negative staphylococci, *Enterococcus, Pseudomonas*
- **Fungal**: *Candida albicans*
- **If bowel integrity compromised**: Gram-negative flora-like *E. coli*
- **Anaerobic** organisms like Bacteroides, Prevotella.

Agents causing burn wound infections: *Staphylococcus aureus, Pseudomonas aeruginosa, Staphylococcus epidermidis.*

LABORATORY DIAGNOSIS OF SKIN AND SOFT TISSUE INFECTIONS

Microscopy

- Gram staining to demonstrate the morphology of causative agent
- KOH mount for fungal infections
- Tzanck smear of vesicle fluid suspected of herpes simplex or Varicella virus infections.

Culture

- **For aerobic bacteria**: Inoculate specimens onto BA, MA, CA
- **For atypical Mycobacteria**: Lowenstein-Jensen medium
- **For fungus**: Sabouraud's dextrose agar
- **For anaerobic bacteria**: Robertson's cooked meat broth, Brain heart infusion broth.

8. STOOL

COMPETENCY
MI3.2: Identify the common etiologic agents of diarrhea and dysentery.
CM3.3: Describe etiology of water borne diseases/jaundice/hepatitis/diarrheal diseases.
IM16.1: Enumerate the indications for stool cultures and blood cultures in patients with acute diarrhea.

Technique of Collection

In a universal container. Stool should be passed into a clean dry container. Pass stool directly into a sterile wide-mouth, leak proof container with a tight fitting lid. Pass stool into a clean, dry bedpan and transfer the stool into a sterile leak proof container with a tight fitting lid.

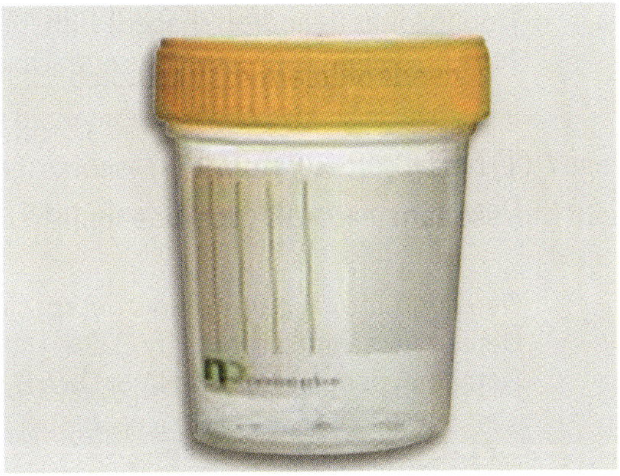

Inoculum Size

Enteric pathogens differ from each other in infective dose

- *Shigella*, enterohemorrhagic *E. coli, Giardia* or *Entamoeba*: 10–100 bacteria or cysts
- *Vibrio cholerae*: 10^5–10^8 bacilli
- *Salmonella*: 10^3–10^5 bacilli.

Enumerate various causes of diarrhea and dysentery and its laboratory diagnosis.

Diarrhea: As per WHO, diarrhea is defined as passage of three or more loose or liquid stools per day, in excess than the usual habitat for that person. Causes are:

- **Bacteria (Enterotoxin mediated):** *Vibrio cholerae, Vibrio parahaemolyticus, Escherichia coli* (Enterotoxigenic), *Clostridium perfringens, Aeromonas* spp.
- ***Cytotoxin mediated:*** *Shigella* spp., enterohemorrhagic *E.coli, Yersinia enterocolitica, Listeria monocytogenes, Clostridum difficile*
- **Neurotoxin mediated:** *Staphylococcus aureus, Bacillus cereus, Clostridium botulinum*
- **Viral:** Rotavirus, norovirus, astrovirus, calicivirus, norwalk virus
- **Parasite:** *Giardia lamblia, Cryptosporidium parvum, Cyclospora, Microsporidia.*

LABORATORY DIAGNOSIS OF ORGANISMS CAUSING DIARRHEA

ORGANISM	PRESENTATION	IDENTIFICATION FEATURES
Vibrio cholerae	Watery diarrhea	Darting motility, Comma-shaped GNB, Catalase (+), Oxidase (+), biochemical reactions MA- Non-lactose fermenting colonies TCBS agar: Sucrose fermenting yellow colored colonies Agglutinates with Vibrio cholerae O1 antisera and Ogawa antisera (common pattern)
Group B Salmonella	Inflammatory diarrhea	Motile, GNB, Catalase (+), Oxidase (-), biochemical reactions MA- Non-lactose fermenting translucent colonies DCA- Non-lactose fermenting colonies with black center XLD- red colonies with black center Agglutinates with Salmonella poly-O antisera and serotype specific antisera
Giardia lamblia	Fatty diarrhea	Trophozoites (tear drop shaped) with four pair of flagella Tetra nucleated oval cyst with central axoneme
Hookworm	Diarrhea	Eggs, oval in shape contains segmented four blastomeres, non-bile stained in stool microscopy
Strongyloides stercoralis	Diarrhea	Detection of rhabditiform larva in stool microscopy
Viral agents (Rotavirus, Norovirus, Adenovirus)	Diarrhea	Detection of viral particles in stool specimen by electron microscopy Detection of viral antigens by ELISA Detection of nucleic acid RNA or DNA by PCR stool specimen

Dysentery

It is characterized by diarrhea with increased blood and mucus, often associated with fever, abdominal pain and tenesmus. Causes are:

- **Bacterial:** Shigella spp. *Campylobacter jejuni,* Enterohemorrhagic *E. coli,* Enterinvasine *E. coli*
- **Parasite:** *Entamoeba histolytica, Balantidium coli.*

LABORATORY DIAGNOSIS OF ORGANISMS CAUSING DYSENTRY

ORGANISM	PRESENTATION	IDENTIFICATION FEATURES
Shigella	Dysentery	Non-motile, GNB, Catalase (+), Oxidase(-), MA- Non lactose fermenting translucent colonies XLD- red colonies without black centre Agglutinates with Shigella polyvalent antisera and specific monovalent antisera
Entamoeba histolytica	Dysentery	Trophozoites or quadrinucleate cysts Detection of specific antigen/genes in stool via PCR

COMPETENCY

MI3.5: Enumerate the causative agents of food poisoning.

CM7.7: Describe and demonstrate the steps in an Investigation of an epidemic of communicable diseases.

In an outbreak of suspected food poisoning, how is the food sample collected and transported to the laboratory? What are the common organisms causing?

Food poisoning refers to an illness acquired through consumption of food and drink contaminated either with microorganisms or their toxins.

During outbreaks vomitus, stool or suspected food materials are the ideal specimens. Food material should be homogenized or washed thoroughly in sterile diluents, e.g. Ringer's solution.

Several non-bacterial agents that can cause food poisoning such as capsaicin , variety of toxins found in fish and shellfish, poisonous mushrooms and some chemical poisons.

Clinical Manifestations and Appearance of Symptoms Within

Bacteria-within 1–6 hours: *Staphylococcus aureus, Bacillus cereus, Clostridium botulinum*

8-16 hours: *Clostridium perfringens, Bacillus cereus*

>16 hours: *Vibrio cholerae,* Enterotoxigenic *E. coli,* Enterohemorrhagic *E. coli,* Salmonella spp., *Campylobacter jejuni,* Shigella spp., *Vibrio parahaemolyticus.*

Purpose of Outbreak Investigation

- To control the current outbreak.
- Prevention of future outbreaks.
- Describe new diseases and learn more about known diseases.
- Evaluation of the effectiveness of prevention programs.
- Evaluation of the effectiveness of the existing surveillance system.
- Training health professionals.
- Responding to public, political, or legal concern.

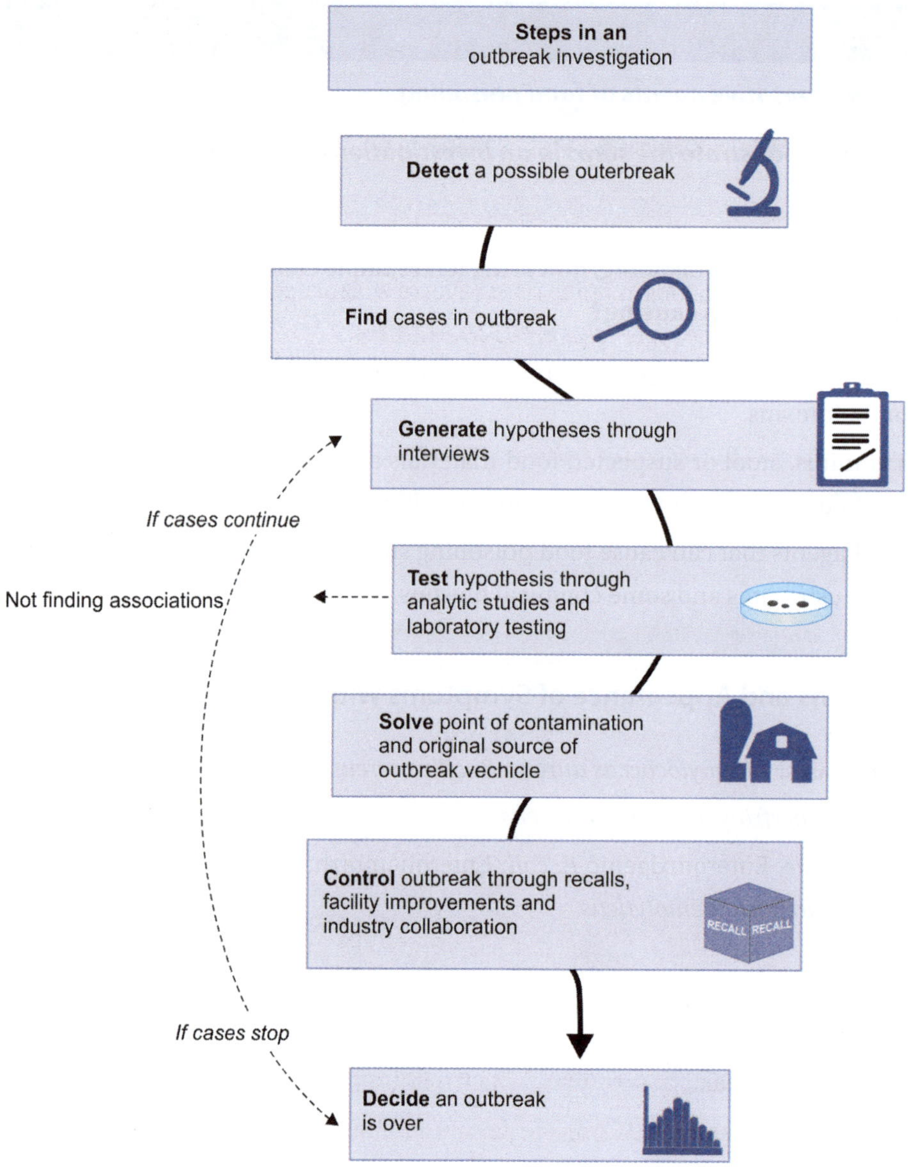
Steps in an outbreak investigation
Detect a possible outerbreak
Find cases in outbreak
Generate hypotheses through interviews
Test hypothesis through analytic studies and laboratory testing
Solve point of contamination and original source of outbreak vechicle
Control outbreak through recalls, facility improvements and industry collaboration
RECALL RECALL
Decide an outbreak is over
If cases continue
Not finding associations
If cases stop

Section 3: Immunology

Chapter 11: Serology

Serology

11
CHAPTER

COMPETENCY
MI1.8: Describe the mechanisms of immunity and response of host immune system to infections.
MI8.15: Choose and interpret the results of laboratory tests used in diagnosis of infectious diseases.

Q1. ENUMERATE THE ANTIGEN-ANTIBODY REACTIONS USED IN SEROLOGICAL DIAGNOSIS.

Types of antigen-antibody reactions.

Conventional Techniques

- Precipitation reaction
- Agglutination reaction
- Complement fixation test
- Neutralization test.

Newer Techniques (Labelled Assays)

- Enzyme-linked immunosorbent assay (ELISA)
- Immunofluorescence assay (IFA)
- Radioimmunoassay (RIA)
- Chemiluminescence-linked immunoassay (CLIA)
- Rapid test: Cassette ELISA, lateral flow test (immunochromatographic test), flow through assay.

Q2. WHAT IS PRECIPITATION AND ENUMERATE VARIOUS PRECIPITATION REACTIONS?

Definition

When a soluble antigen reacts with its specific antibody in the presence of an electrolyte at optimal temperature and pH, it leads to formation of antigen-antibody complex in the form of:

- Insoluble precipitate band when gel containing medium is used or insoluble floccules or precipitate ring when liquid medium is used.
- **Precipitation in liquid medium**
  - Ring test: Ascoli's thermoprecipitin test, Streptococcal grouping by Lancefield's technique
  - Slide test: Flocculation test - VDRL test for syphilis
  - Tube test: Kahn's test for syphilis
- **Precipitation in gel (immunodiffusion)**
  - Single diffusion in one dimension (Oudin procedure)
  - Double diffusion in one dimension (Oakley Fultrope procedure)
  - Single diffusion in two dimensions (Radial immunodiffusion)
  - Double diffusion in two dimensions (Ouchterlony procedure)
- **Immunoelectrophoresis**
- **Electroimmunodiffusion**
  - Countercurrent immunoelectrophoresis (CIEP)
  - Rocket electrophoresis.

Q3. DEFINE AGGLUTINATION AND ENUMERATE VARIOUS AGGLUTINATION REACTIONS.

Definition

When a particulate or insoluble antigen is mixed with its specific antibody in the presence of electrolytes at a suitable temperature and pH, particles are clumped or agglutinated.

1. Direct Agglutination Test

- Slide agglutination test: For blood grouping and cross matching
- Tube agglutination test: Widal test for Enteric fever
  - Hetrophile agglutination test: Weil-Felix for typhus fever, Paul Bunnel test for infectious mononucleosis
- Microscopic agglutination: For leptospirosis.

2. Passive Agglutination Test (For Antibody Detection)

A precipitation reaction can be converted into agglutination test by attaching soluble antigens to the surface of carrier such as latex particles, bentonite and red blood cells.

- Latex agglutination test (LAT)—for detection of ASO (antistreptolysin antibody), CRP, RA
- Indirect hemagglutination test.

3. Reverse Passive Agglutination Reaction

When instead of antigen, antibody is absorbed on the carrier particles for estimation of antigens.

- Coagglutination test: *Staphylococcus aureus* (protein A) acts as a carrier molecule. Specific antibody binds with Fc portion and Fab site remain free. Such sensitized cells are used for detection of antigen, e.g., Salmonella typhi antigen in serum.
- For detection of hepatitis B surface antigen (HBsAg).

Q4. DESCRIBE THE PRINCIPLE AND APPLICATIONS OF COOMBS TEST.

It is performed to diagnose Rh incompatibility by detecting Rh antibody from mother's and baby's serum. It is used to test for autoimmune hemolytic anemia.

Direct Coombs test (also known as the direct antiglobulin test or DAT) is used to detect if antibodies have bound to RBC surface antigens in vivo. A blood sample is taken and the RBCs are washed and then incubated with antihuman globulin. If this produces agglutination of RBCs, the direct Coombs test is **positive, e.g., erythroblastosis fetalis**.

Indirect Coombs test (also known as the indirect antiglobulin test or IAT) is used to detect **in vitro** antibody-antigen reactions. It is used to detect very low concentrations of antibodies present in a patient's plasma/serum prior to a blood transfusion. In antenatal care, this test is used to screen pregnant women for antibodies that may cause hemolytic disease of the newborn. The IAT can also be used for compatibility testing, antibody identification.

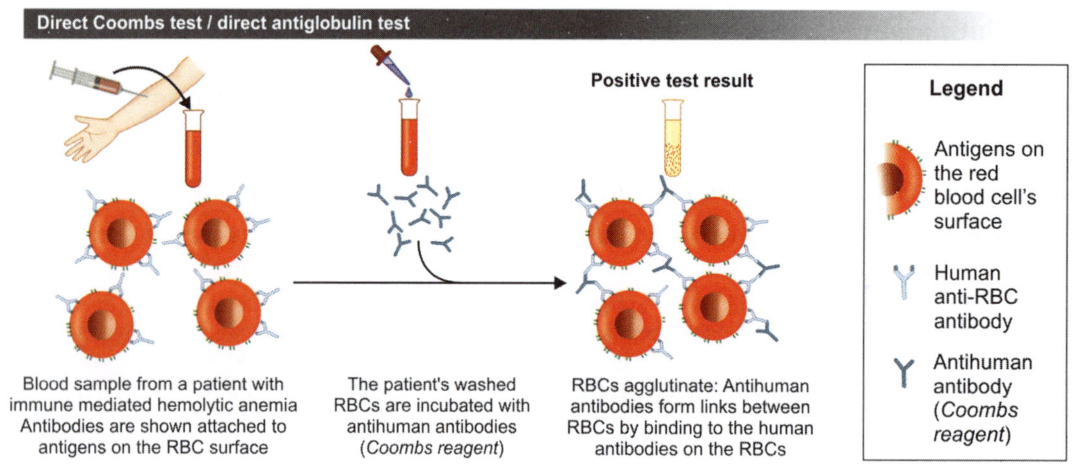

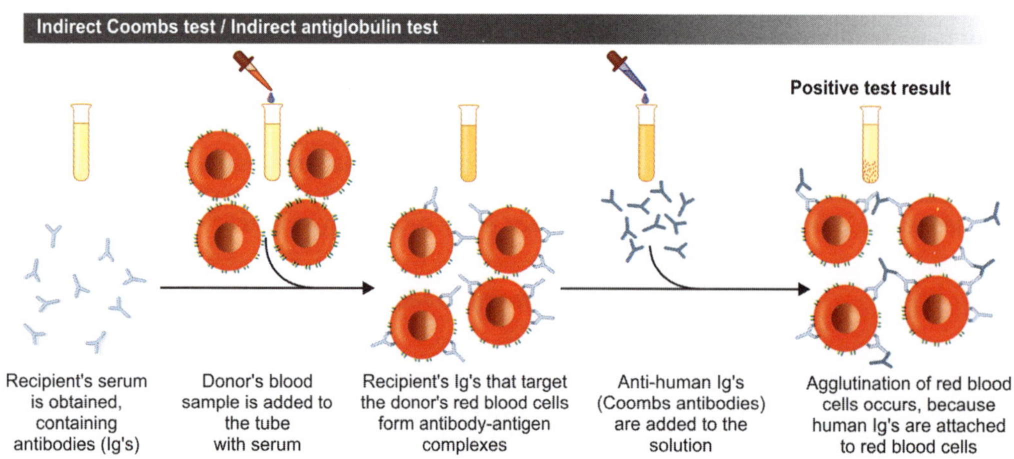

Q.5 WRITE BRIEFLY ABOUT COMPLEMENT FIXATION TEST.

Principle: It is a two way step. When antigen and antibodies are mixed, complement is fixed to the antigen-antibody complex. It can be detected by adding amboreceptors (Sheep RBCs coated with anti-sheep RBC antibody).

First Step

Antigen (soluble or particulate) + test serum + guinea pig complement are all added together.

- ***If the test serum is positive for antibody***—Ag-Ab complex is formed. Complement gets fixed to the complex, so there will be no free complements in the serum.
- ***If the test serum is negative for antibody***—there is no Ag-Ab complex. Complements are not fixed, hence remain free in the serum.

Second Step

A hemolysis indicator system is added. It consists of sheep RBCs coated with its antibodies called amboreceptors.

- ***If the test serum is positive for antibody***—no free complement in serum for binding to amboreceptors—***no hemolysis***.
- ***If the test serum is negative for antibody***—free complement attached to amboreceptors bound on sheep RBCs—***hemolysis***.

Q6. WHAT IS IMMUNOFLUORESCENCE AND DESCRIBE ITS TECHNIQUES? MENTION THEIR APPLICATIONS.

Principle: Fluorescence refers to absorbing high energy-shorter wavelength ultraviolet light rays by the fluorescent compounds and in turn emitting visible light rays with a low energy longer wavelength. Commonly used fluorescent dyes are fluorescein isothiocyanate, rhodamine.

Types of Immunofluorescence Tests

Direct immunofluorescence test: Specific antibodies tagged with fluorescent dye are used for detection of unknown antigen. If antigen is present, it reacts with labeled antibodies and fluorescence can be observed.

Indirect immunofluorescence assay: A known antigen is fixed on slide and unknown antibody in patient's serum attaches to the known antigen on the slide. For detection of antigen antibody reaction, fluorescein tagged antibody to human globulin is added, thus which is observed under fluorescent microscope.

Applications

Detection of autoantibodies (antinuclear antibody) in autoimmune diseases.

Detection of bacteria in blood, CSF, urine, feces, tissue and other specimens.

Detection of microbial antigens—rabies antigen in corneal smear.

Detection of viral antigens in cell lines inoculated with the specimens.

Q7. WRITE BRIEFLY ABOUT RADIOIMMUNOASSAY (RIA). HOW IS RADIOIMMUNOASSAY USEFUL IN DIAGNOSIS?

Radioimmunoassay (RIA) is an immunoassay that is based on competition for a fixed amounts of specific antibody between a known radiolabeled antigen and unknown unlabelled (test) antigen. After antigen- antibody reaction, antigen is separated into 'free' and 'bound' fractions and their radioactivity is measured.

It uses radiolabeled molecules in a stepwise formation of immune complexes. An RIA is a very sensitive in vitro assay technique used to measure concentrations of substances, usually measuring antigen concentrations.

USES

- The test can be used to determine very small quantities (e.g. nanogram) of antigens and antibodies in the serum.
- The test is used for quantitation of hormones, drugs, HBsAg, and other viral antigens.
- Analyze nanomolar and picomolar concentrations of hormones in biological fluids.

Q8. MENTION THE PRINCIPLE OF ELISA. DESCRIBE THE DIFFERENT TYPES OF ELISA DONE. LIST OUT THE VARIOUS APPLICATIONS.

Principle: ELISA can provide a useful measurement of antigen or antibody concentration.

There are two components:

1. **Immunosorbent:** An absorbing material (polyvinyl, polystyrene) is used that specifically absorbs the known antigen or antibody present in serum.
2. **Enzyme:** Is used to label one of the components of immunoassay.

Following antigen- antibody reaction , chromogenic substrate specific to enzyme (o-phenylenediamine for peroxidase and p-nitrophenyl phosphate for alkaline phosphatase) is added. Reaction is detected by reading optical density. **(Ag + AB complex) - enzyme + substrate → activates the chromogen → color change → Detected by spectrophotometry.**

Types of ELISA

Direct ELISA: Used for detection of antigen

Indirect ELISA: Used for detection of antibody/antigen

Sandwich ELISA: Used for detection of antigen - direct (single Ab) and indirect (double Ab)

Competitive ELISA: Used for detection of antigen/antibody

Cassette ELISA (Cylinder ELISA): Used for detection of antibody.

Applications

- **For antigen detection:** Hepatitis B surface antigen, hepatitis B inner core antigen, NS1 dengue antigen
- **For antibody detection:** Hepatitis B, C, HIV, dengue, Epstein-Barr virus, Herpes Simplex virus, toxoplasmosis, leishmaniasis.

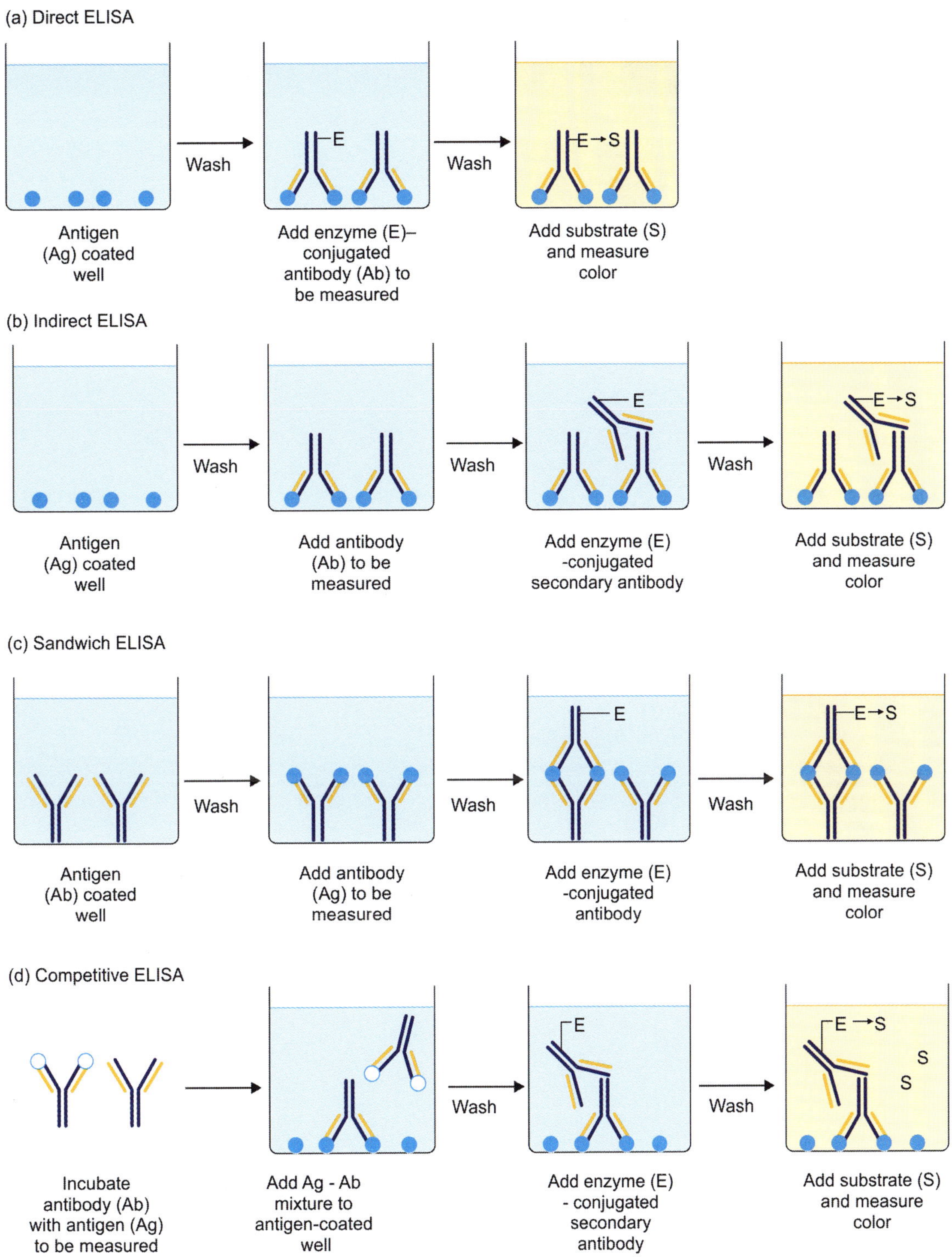

Types of ELISA

Section 4: Parasitology

Stool Examination

12
CHAPTER

COMPETENCY
MI1.2: Perform and identify the different causative agents of Infectious diseases by stool routine microscope.
MI3.2: Identify the common etiologic agents of diarrhea and dysentery.
IM16.9: Identify common parasitic causes of diarrhea under the microscope in a stool examination.
CM3.3: Describe etiology of water borne diseases/diarrheal diseases.

Aim

To do a microscopic examination of the given sample of stool and report.

Requirement

Normal saline, Lugol's iodine, glass slides, cover slips, compound microscope, stool suspension.

Composition of Lugol's Iodine

- Iodine crystals : 1 g
- Potassium iodine : 2 g
- Distilled water : 100 mL.

Procedure

- A drop of normal saline is placed on the center of a clean slide.
- About 2 mg of the given sample of stool is emulsified in the saline.
- A cover slip is then placed on the emulsion avoiding air bubbles.
- After reducing the light by lowering the condenser and using the concave mirror, the preparations first screened under low power.
- When a cyst or an ovum is seen the details are observed by focussing under high power.
- If cysts are seen, another preparation is made by emulsifying about 3 mg of stool sample in Lugol's Iodine. This helps to stain the nuclei.

Advantages of Iodine

- Lugol's iodine stain is intended to be used with wet mount preparations and concentration techniques for the detection of intestinal protozoa
- Lugol's iodine is a rapid, non-specific contrast dye that is added to direct wet mounts of fecal material to aid in differentiating parasitic cysts from host white blood cells.
- Iodine stains protozoan nuclei and intracytoplasmic organelles as brown, making them easier to identify. It paralyzes the motility of organisms and may hinder some parasitic structures.

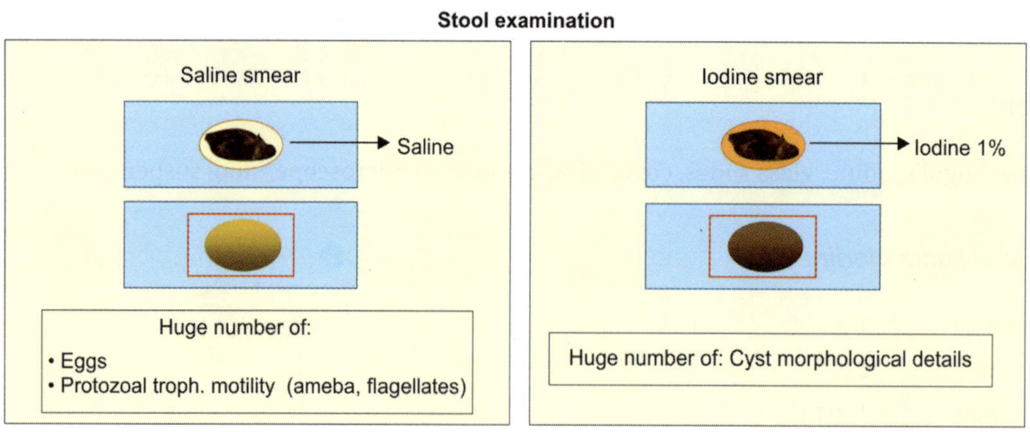

Morphology of Various Parasites

13
CHAPTER

COMPETENCY

MI3.2: Identify the common etiologic agents of diarrhea and dysentery.

IM16.9: Identify common parasitic causes of diarrhea under the microscope in a stool examination.

CM3.3: Describe etiology of water borne diseases/diarrheal diseases.

1. Cyst of *Entamoeba histolytica*

- Quadrinucleate cyst, measures 18-40 µm in size
- Surrounded by thick chitinous wall
- 1-4 chromatid bars are present
- Cysts are present in lumen of colon and formed feces.

2. Cyst of *Giardia lamblia*

- Lives in duodenum and upper jejunum
- Oval ellipsoidal in shape with thick cyst wall
- Bilaterally symmetrical with two axostyles placed diagonally
- Two pairs of nuclei are also present
- Demonstration by Enterotest.

3. *Taenia saginata*

- Large, 5–10 meters in length
- Scolex is rhomboidal
- 2 mm in diameter
- Four suckers are present, pigmented
- Lacks rostellum and hooklets
- Bile-stained ova seen.

4. *Taenia solium*

- Small, 2–3 meters in length, globular
- Possess rostellum and hooklets
- Suckers are not pigmented
- Bile-stained ova.

5. Ovum of *Hymenolepis nana*

- Oval 30–45 μm in size
- Non-bile stained
- Outer membrane is thin colorless, inner membrane (embryophore) encloses oncosphere
- 3 pairs of hooklets.

6. Fertilized Egg of *Ascaris lumbricoides*

- Round to oval in shape, 60–75 µm in size
- Bile stained
- Surrounded by thick, transparent shell, consisting of vitelline membrane
- Outermost layer is coarsely, regular, albuminoid.

7. Unfertilized Egg of *Ascaris lumbricoides*

- Narrower and longer, 90 × 55 µm in size
- Bile stained
- Egg contains small atrophied ovum with thin shell within an irregular coating of albumin
- Heaviest of helminthic egg, do not float in saturated solution of common salt.

8. Egg of *Ancylostoma duodenale*

- Oval and elliptical , 60 × 40 µm in size
- Non-bile stained
- Possess a segmented ovum with four blastomeres
- Clear space between the segmented ovum and egg shell.

9. Egg of *Enterobius vermicularis*

- Non-bile stained
- Embryonated egg is the infective stage
- Egg shell is thin, hyaline, transparent, encloses larva.

10. Trypanosomes

- Morphological forms—tyrpomastigote and amastigote
- Trypomastigote is infective form found in peripheral blood, C-shaped 20 μm in size
- Kinetoplast is situated in the posterior end
- Stained by Giemsa and Wright stains
- Undulating membrane is present.

11. *Leishmania donovani*

- Morphological forms: LD bodies and promastigotes
- Promastigote: Cells are elongated, posterior end is pointed
- Long flagellum projects from posterior end
- Amastigote form: Resides in reticuloendothelial system, is oval body measuring 2–4 μm in size. Can be stained by Wright and Giemsa stain.

COMPETENCY

MI2.6: Identify the causative agent of Malaria and Filariasis.

IMP4.15: Perform and interpret a malarial smear.

Causative organism for malaria: *Plasmodium falciparum, P. vivax, P. malariae, P. ovale, P. knowlesi.*

Different stains used are: Giemsa, Leishman, Romanowsky, Wright's and Jaswant Singh Bhattacharya stain

- Thick smear: For identification of malaria.
- Thin smear: For species identification.
- Occurrence of multiple rings with accole formation: Banana shaped gametocytes, diagnostic of *P. falciparum.*

Malarial Smear

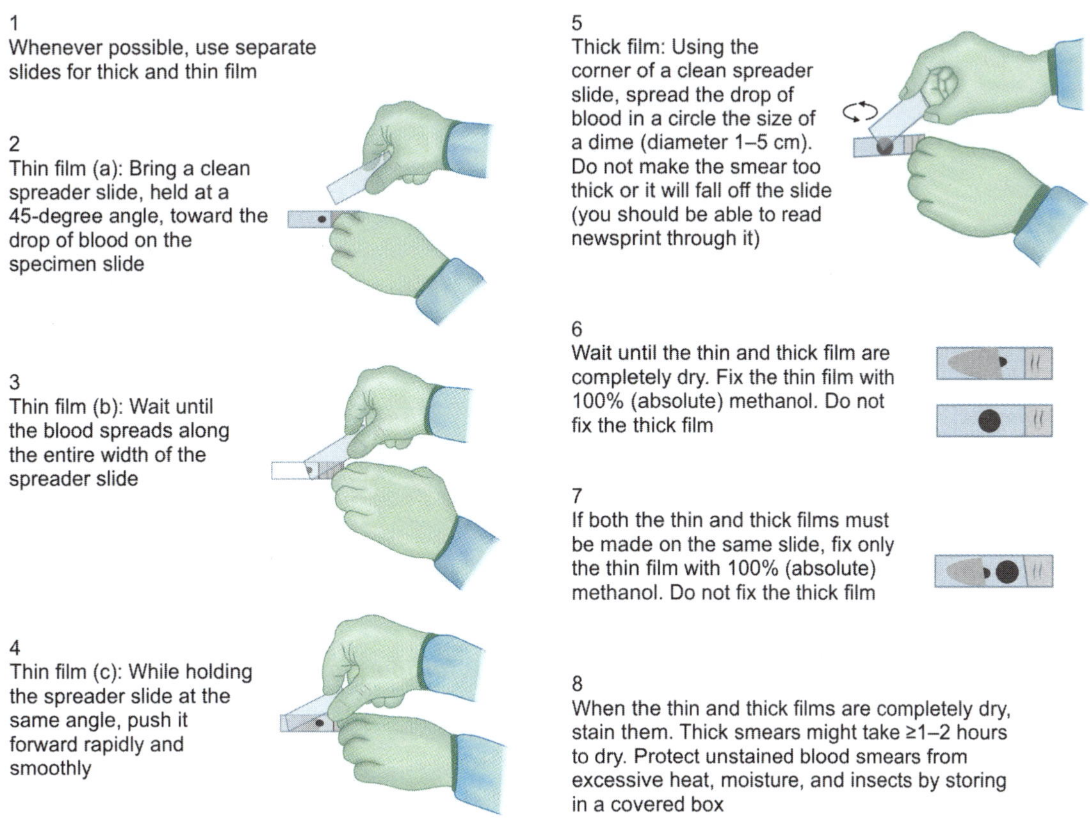

1
Whenever possible, use separate slides for thick and thin film
2
Thin film (a): Bring a clean spreader slide, held at a 45-degree angle, toward the drop of blood on the specimen slide
3
Thin film (b): Wait until the blood spreads along the entire width of the spreader slide
4
Thin film (c): While holding the spreader slide at the same angle, push it forward rapidly and smoothly
5
Thick film: Using the corner of a clean spreader slide, spread the drop of blood in a circle the size of a dime (diameter 1–5 cm). Do not make the smear too thick or it will fall off the slide (you should be able to read newsprint through it)
6
Wait until the thin and thick film are completely dry. Fix the thin film with 100% (absolute) methanol. Do not fix the thick film
7
If both the thin and thick films must be made on the same slide, fix only the thin film with 100% (absolute) methanol. Do not fix the thick film
8
When the thin and thick films are completely dry, stain them. Thick smears might take ≥1–2 hours to dry. Protect unstained blood smears from excessive heat, moisture, and insects by storing in a covered box

Quantitative Buffy Coat

Acridine orange (AO) binds deoxyribonucleic acids and ribonucleic acids. The malaria parasite binds acridine orange in the nucleus and the cytoplasm and emits green and red fluorescence when excited at 480 nm allowing the detection and examination of parasite morphology by fluorescent microscopy.

Rapid diagnostic tests: RDTs for detection of antigen. Antigens targeted by RDTs are:

- Histidine rich protein-II (HRP-II)
- Parasite lactate dehydrogenase (pLDH)
- Aldolase.

Complications

Anemia, hemoglobinuria, hemoglobinemia, blackwater fever, acute renal failure, tropical splenomegaly, cerebral malaria, hypoglycemia.

Draw malarial smear for *P. falciparum*

FILARIA

Causative agent for filariasis: *Wuchereria bancrofti*

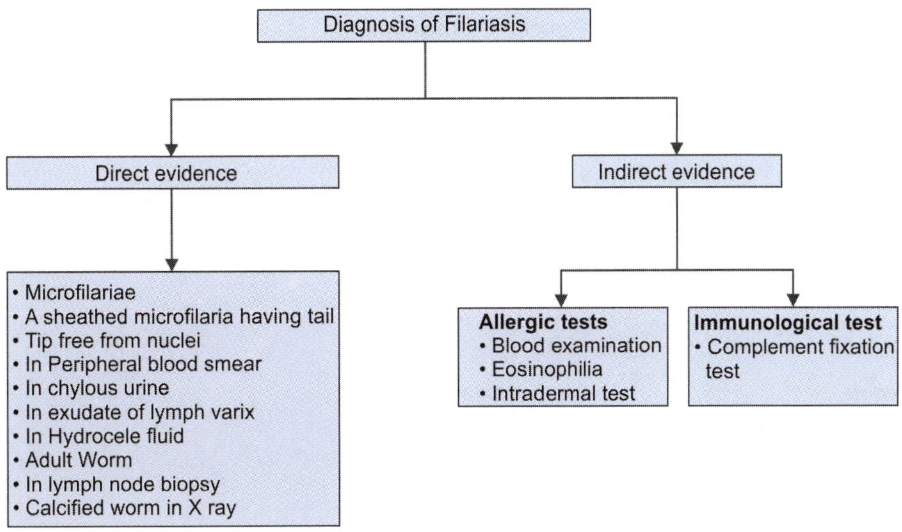

Mention the infective forms of the following protozoans.

PROTOZOAN	INFECTIVE FORMS
Entamoeba histolytica	Tetranucleate cyst
Naegleria fowleri	Trophozoite
Acanthamoeba nigricans	Trophozoite and cyst
Glardia lamblia	Cyst
Trichomonas vaginalis	Trophozoite
Leishmania	Promastigote
Balantidium coli	Cyst
Plasmodium	Sporozoite
Toxoplasma gondii	Oocyst
Cryptosporidium	Oocyst and tissue cyst

Mention the infective forms of the following helminths.

HELMINTH	INFECTIVE FORM
Taenia	Cysticercus bovis (*T. saginata*) and Cysticercus cellulosae (*T. solium*)
Diphyllobothrum latum	Pleucocercoid larvae
Echinococcus granulosus	Egg
Hymenolepis nana	Egg
Fasciola	Metacercaria larva
Paragonimus westermani	Metacercaria larva
Schistosoma	Cercaria larva
Ascaris lumbricoides	Egg
Ankylostoma duodenale	Filariform larva
Trichinella spiralis	Encysted larva
Strongyloides stercoralis	Filariform larva
Trichuris trichiura	Egg
Enterobius vermicularis	Egg
Filarial worms	3rd stage larva
Dracunculus medinensis	3rd stage larva

Define

(a) Viviparous parasites. Give examples.

(b) Ovo-viviparous parasite. Give example.

(c) Oviparous parasites. Give examples.

Section 5: Mycology

Chapter 14: Morphology of Fungi

Morphology of Fungi

14

CHAPTER

COMPETENCY

MI1.1: Describe the different causative agents of infectious diseases, methods of detection of microbes in health and disease.

MI1.2: Perform and identify the different causative agents of infectious diseases by KOH, India Ink, LPCB mount.

Aim: To make a lactophenol cotton blue preparation of the given fungal culture and report.

Requirements: Lactophenol cotton blue (LPCB) solution.

Composition of Lactophenol Cotton Blue

- Phenol crystals : 20 g
- Lactic acid : 20 mL
- Glycerol : 40 mL
- Distilled water : 20 mL
- Cotton blue : 0.075 g

The phenol crystals are dissolved in the liquid by gently warming. Add dye to it.

Procedure

- A drop of lactophenol cotton blue is placed on the center of a clean slide.
- Using a sterile needle, a small portion of the pure fungal colony in the given culture is transferred to the drop of LCB slide.
- It is then teased apart with dissecting needles.
- A cover slip is carefully placed on the preparation avoiding air bubbles.
- After reducing the light, by lowering the condenser and using the concave mirror, the preparation is first screened under low power to visualize the hyphae and the conidia
- It is then visualized under high power in order to identify the fungus.

KOH Mount

Potassium hydroxide (KOH) mount is a very useful test for the laboratory diagnosis of fungal infection of tissues especially skin, hair and nails. KOH separates the fungal elements from intact cells as it digests the protein debris and dissolves cement substances that holds the keratinized cells together and makes it easy to visualize under the microscope.

Requirements

- 10% KOH
- Coverslip
- Glass slide
- Needle
- Bunsen flame
- Specimen.

KOH Procedure

- Place the specimens like epidermal scales, nail, hair, skin scraping or tissue on a clean glass slide.
- Pour a drop of 10% KOH on the specimen and place a coverslip over it.
- Heat the slide gently over flame.
- Leave the slide for 5–10 minutes.
- Examine the slide under microscope.

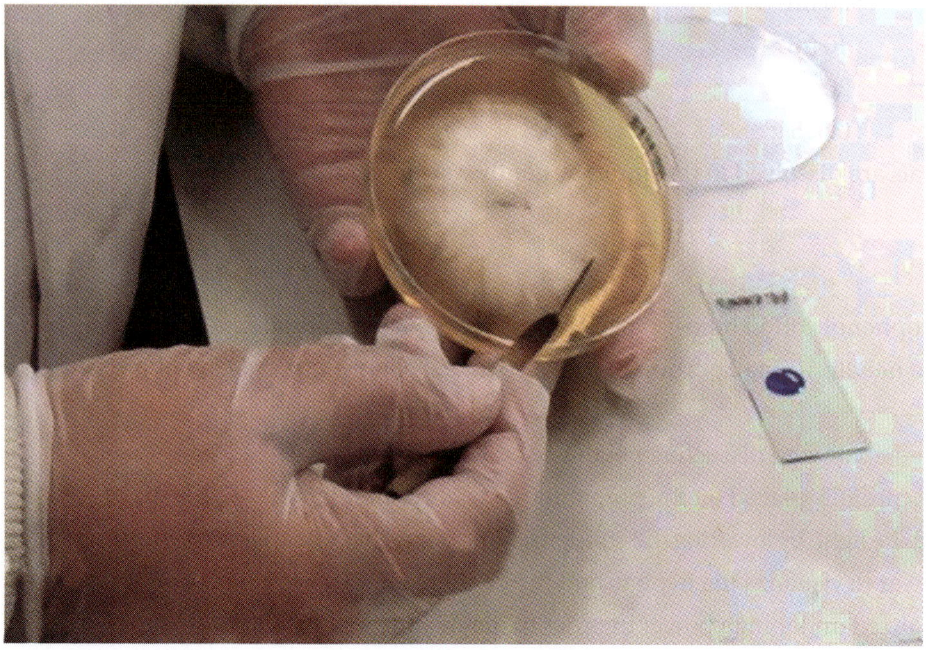

1. *Cryptococcus neoformans*

- Capsulated yeast cell
- Demonstration of capsule by—negative staining by India ink
- Causes opportunistic infection Cryptococcosis
- CSF sample is taken.

2. DR7.2: Identify *Candida* spp. in fungal scrapings and KOH

- Ovoid or spherical budding yeast cells are seen on gram staining
- Pseudohyphae—tube like elongations seen in tissue for invasion.
- Can cause opportunistic infections
- Germ tube test or Reynolds-Braude phenomenon is seen.

3. *Trichophyton*

- Segmented hyphae with conidia are seen on lactophenol cotton blue (LPCB) stain
- Microconidia—abundant, arranged along hyphae in *T. rubrum*
- Macroconidia—scanty with blunt edges
- Infects skin, hair and nail.

4. *Microsporum*

- Segmented hyphae
- Microconidia are few and plenty of macroconidia are present
- Macroconidia: Large, multicellular, spindle shaped
- Infects skin and hair.

5. *Epidermophyton*

- Microconidia are absent
- Macroconidia are abundant- multicellular, pear shaped
- Infects skin and nails.

6. *Madurella mycetomatis*

- Pus from sinuses containing granules or grains is processed
- Granules—microcolonies of fungus
- LCB mount of crushed granules.

7. *Rhinosporidium*

- Large number of fungal spherules are seen
- Each spherule matures into a sporangium 350 µm in size
- Thousands of endospores (6–9 µm) in each sporangium
- *Rhinosporidium seeberi*—mainly seen as nasal mass.

8. *Aspergillus niger*

- Grossly, colonies are black in color
- Septate hyphae with conidiophores are seen
- Vesicle is globular with uniseriate/biseriate sterigmata.

9. *Aspergillus fumigatus*

- Grossly colonies are dark green in color
- Vesicle is conical in shape with uniseriate sterigmata
- Septate hyphae with conidiophores are seen.

10. *Penicillium*

- Grossly colonies are blue-green in color with white border and a powdery surface
- Septate hyphae with branched conidiophores, with two rows of sterigmata bearing chain of spores—brush or broom appearance.

11. *Mucor*

- Broad aseptate hyphae are seen
- Sporangiophores are seen with sporangia and spores
- Rhizoids are absent.

12. *Rhizopus*

- Broad aseptate hyphae are seen
- Rhizoids are present.

Various specimens, possible fungal pathogens and their methods of demonstration in the following clinical conditions:

DISEASE	SPECIMEN	POSSIBLE FUNGAL PATHOGENS	METHOD OF DEMONSTRATION
Dermatophytosis	Skin, hair and nail		
Meningitis	CSF		
Keratomycosis	Corneal scrapings		
Otomycosis	Ear swab		
Nasal polyps	Nasal mucosa scrapings		
Resp. tract infection	Sputum		
Vaginitis	Vaginal swab		
Mycetoma	Pus with granules		
Systemic mycoses	Sputum, bone marrow biopsy, blood		

Section 6: Virology

Morphology of Viruses

15
CHAPTER

COMPETENCY

MI1.1: Describe the different causative agents of infectious diseases, methods of detection of microbes in health and disease.

1. Herpes virus

- Icosahedral symmetry, 150-200 nm in diameter
- Lipid envelope with peplomers
- Tegument present between capsid and peplomers
- ***Tzanck cells*** (multinucleated giant cells with faceted nuclei and homogeneously stained ground glass chromatic) in HSV-2.

2. Adenovirus

- Non-enveloped, 70-90 nm in diameter
- Icosahedral in symmetry with 252 capsomers
- Fiber protein projecting from each vertex-space vehicle appearance
- Causes respiratory tract infections.

3. Picornavirus

- Non-enveloped virus, spherical shaped
- Icosahedral capsid, 60 capsomers present
- Each capsid has 4 viral proteins, possess ssRNA
- Contains Enterovirus (Polio virus) and Rhinovirus.

4. Rhabdovirus

- Bullet shaped virus with one end rounded and other end flat (75 nm ×180 nm)
- Lipoprotein envelope with hemagglutinin spikes
- M layer present lines the envelope
- Nucleocapsid has helical symmetry, has ss negative sense RNA.

COMPETENCY

MI2.7, IM6.4: Describe epidemiology, etiopathogenesis, evolution, complication, opportunistic infections, diagnosis, prevention and principles of management of HIV.

DR11.1: Describe etiology, pathogenesis, clinical features of dermatologic manifestations of HIV and its complications including opportunistic infections.

IM6.2: Define and classify HIV AIDS based on CDC criteria.

IM6.10: Choose and interpret appropriate diagnostic tests to diagnose and classify severity of HIV-AIDS including specific tests of HIV.

Definition of HIV Infection

Adults and Children 18 Months or Older

HIV infection is diagnosed based on: Positive HIV antibody testing (rapid or laboratory-based enzyme immunoassay). This is usually confirmed by two more HIV antibody test (rapid or laboratory-based enzyme immunoassay) relying on different antigens or of different operating characteristics.

Children Younger than 18 Months

HIV infection is diagnosed based on: A positive virological test for HIV or its components (HIV-RNA or HIV-DNA or ultrasensitive HIV p24 antigen) confirmed by a second virological test obtained from a separate determination taken more than four weeks after birth.

Positive antibody testing is not recommended for definitive or confirmatory diagnosis of HIV infection in children until 18 months of age.

Characteristic Features of HIV

80–110 nm in size, enveloped virus. Envelope is made up of:

- ***Lipid part:*** Host cell membrane derived
- ***Protein part:*** Glycoprotein 120 (gp-120) and Glycoprotein 41 (gp-41)
- ***Nucleocapsid:*** Icosahedral in symmetry, made up of core protein, Inner core encloses two identical copies of ss positive linear RNA.

WHO CLINICAL STAGING OF HIV/AIDS FOR ADULTS AND ADOLESCENTS WITH CONFIRMED HIV INFECTION

Clinical Stage 1

- Asymptomatic
- Persistent generalized lymphadenopathy.

Clinical Stage 2

- Unexplained moderate weight loss (<10% of presumed or measured body weight)
- Recurrent respiratory tract infections (sinusitis, tonsillitis, otitis media and pharyngitis)
- Herpes zoster
- Angular cheilitis
- Recurrent oral ulceration
- Papular pruritic eruptions
- Seborrheic dermatitis
- Fungal nail infections.

Clinical Stage 3

- Unexplained severe weight loss (>10% of presumed or measured body weight)
- Unexplained chronic diarrhea for longer than one month
- Unexplained persistent fever (above 37.5°C intermittent or constant for longer than one month)
- Persistent oral candidiasis
- Oral hairy leukoplakia
- Pulmonary tuberculosis
- Severe bacterial infections (such as pneumonia, empyema, pyomyositis, bone or joint infection, meningitis or bacteremia)
- Acute necrotizing ulcerative stomatitis, gingivitis or periodontitis
- Unexplained anemia (<8 g/dL), neutropenia (<0.5 × 109 per liter) and/or chronic thrombocytopenia (<50 × 109 per liter)

Clinical Stage 4

- HIV wasting syndrome
- Pneumocystis pneumonia
- Recurrent severe bacterial pneumonia
- Chronic herpes simplex infection (orolabial, genital or anorectal of more than one month's duration or visceral at any site)

- Esophageal candidiasis (or candidiasis of trachea, bronchi or lungs)
- Extrapulmonary tuberculosis
- Kaposi's sarcoma
- Cytomegalovirus infection (retinitis or infection of other organs)
- Central nervous system toxoplasmosis
- HIV encephalopathy
- Extrapulmonary cryptococcosis including meningitis
- Disseminated non-tuberculous mycobacterial infection
- Progressive multifocal leukoencephalopathy
- Chronic cryptosporidiosis
- Chronic isosporiasis
- Disseminated mycosis (extrapulmonary histoplasmosis or coccidioidomycosis)
- Recurrent septicemia (including non-typhoidal *Salmonella*)
- Lymphoma (cerebral or B-cell non-Hodgkin)
- Invasive cervical carcinoma
- Atypical disseminated leishmaniasis
- Symptomatic HIV-associated nephropathy or symptomatic HIV-associated cardiomyopathy.

LABORATORY DIAGNOSIS

- **Screening tests** (ERS) (antibody detection): ELISA/Rapid test/Simple test
- **Supplemental tests** (antibody detection): Western blot, immunofluorescence, radio-immuno-precipitation assay
- **Confirmatory tests:**
  - p24 antigen detection
  - Viral culture
  - HIV RNA by reverse transcriptase-PCR, real-time PCR for estimating viral load
  - Branched DNA assay
  - Nucleic acid sequence based amplification (NASBA)
  - HIV DNA testing for pediatric patients is confirmatory test.

Non-specific Tests for HIV Detection

- Low CD4 T cell count
- Hypergammaglobulinemia
- Altered CD4:CD8 ratio.

COMPETENCY

MI3.7: Describe epidemiology, etiopathogenesis and discuss viral markers in the evolution of viral hepatitis. Discuss the modalities in diagnosis and prevention of viral hepatitis.

MI3.8: Choose the appropriate laboratory test in the diagnosis of viral hepatitis with emphasis on viral markers.

IM5.4: Describe and discuss the epidemiology, microbiology and clinical evolution of infective viral hepatitis.

Morphology of Hepatitis B

Particles seen on electron microscope are:

- Abundant spherical particles of 20 nm in diameter
- Tubular particles: 200 nm in diameter
- Double shelled particle: Dane particle - 42 nm in size, spherical.

Serological Testings Done

Immunochromatographic tests, ELISA can be done

- Antigen markers: HBsAg, HBeAg, HBcAg
- Antibody marker: Anti-HBs, anti-HBE and anti-HBc
- Molecular markers: HBV DNA
- Non-specific markers: Elevated liver enzymes and serum bilirubin.

TEST	POSITIVE RESULT INDICATES
➢ ALT elevation	➢ Hepatocyte injury and can occur in acute or chronic hepatitis and other types of liver disease. Patients with severe cirrhosis may have ALT levels within the normal range
➢ Anti-HAV IgM	➢ Acute hepatitis A infection NB given the low prevalence of HAV infections in BC, many anti-HAV IgM positive results may reflect false positivity - clinical correlation is required
➢ Anti-HAV total or anti-HAV IgG	➢ If the anti-HAV IgM is non-reactive, a positive result indicates immunity to hepatitis A from natural infection or vaccination
➢ HBsAg	➢ Hepatisis B virus infection and infectiousness
➢ Anti-HBc IgM	➢ Acute or chronic hepatitis B infection. Rarely required for clinical management. About 20% of chronic HBV infected people display anti-HBc IgM
➢ Anti-HBc total	➢ Antibody to this marker does not imply immunity
➢ Anti-HBs	➢ Immunity to hepatitis B, due to vaccination or natural infection. If both anti-HBc total and anti-HBc reactive (and HBsAg is non-reactive) this indicates a resolved hepatitis B infection
➢ HBeAg, anti-HBe, HBV DNA	➢ These tests are sued to assess disease severity or for treatment eligibility/monitoring and should not be ordered for routine diagnosis
➢ Anti-HCV	➢ Indicates exposure to hepatitis C. Does not imply immunity, usually represents active infection confirm status by testing for HCV RNA
➢ HCV RNA	➢ Presence of hepatitis C virus infection

Prophylaxis

- Recombinant subunit vaccine (3 doses-0,1 and 6 months)
- Hepatitis B Immunoglobin (HBIG): 0.05–0.07 mL/kg body weight.

Complications of Serum Hepatitis

Hepatocellular carcinoma, cirrhosis, arthralgia, urticaria, polyarthritis, glomerulonephritis.

Cultivation and Identification of Viruses

16
CHAPTER

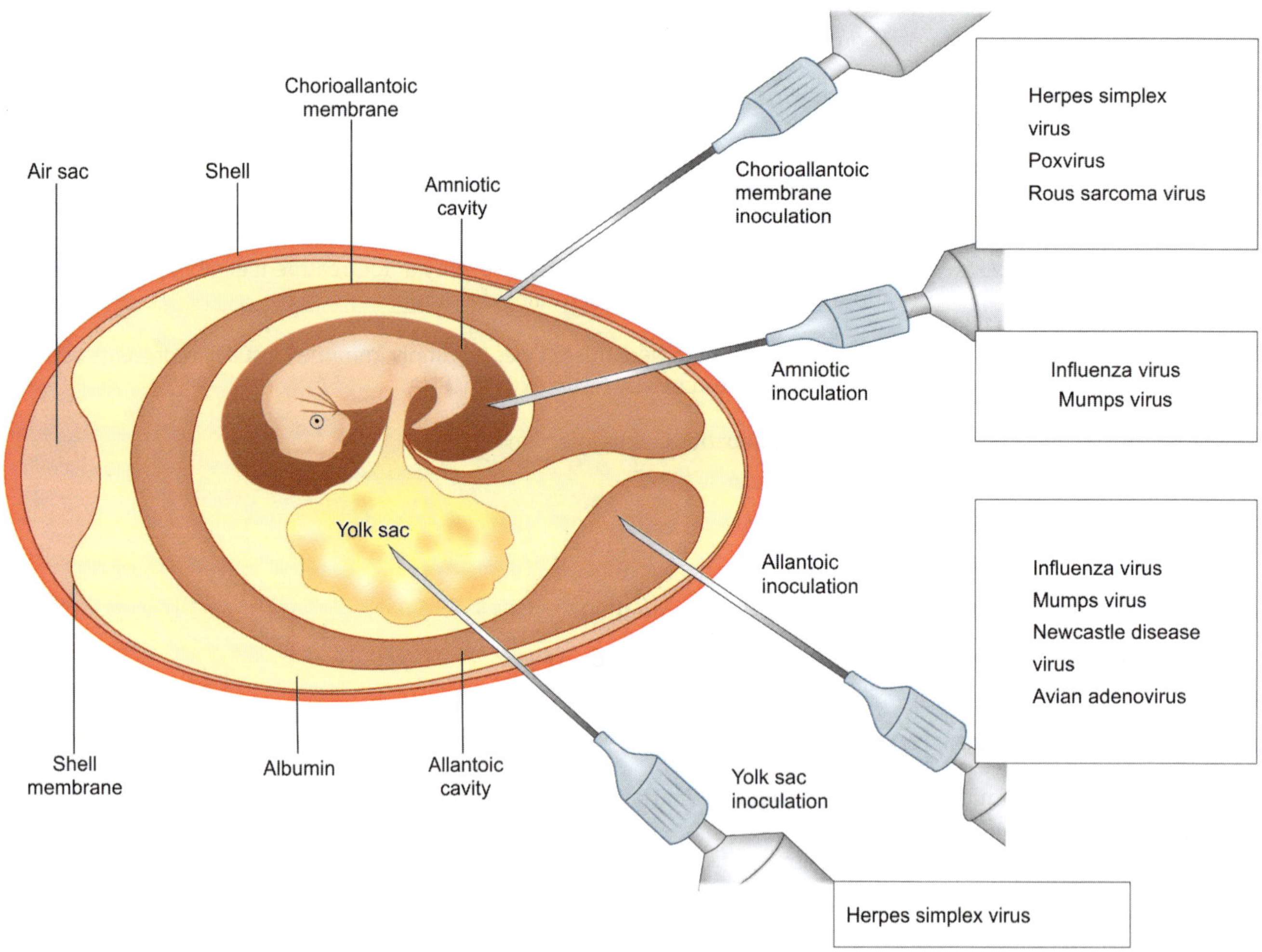

Growth of viruses in embryonated egg:
An embryonated chicken egg showing the different compartments in which viruses may grow. The different routes by which viruses are inoculated into eggs are indicated.

SPECIMENS OBTAINED FOR THE ISOLATION OF VIRUSES IN THE LABORATORY

MI1.1: Describe the different causative agents if infectious diseases, methods used in their detection.

MI6.2: Identify common etiologic agents of upper respiratory tract infections.

MI6.3: Identify common etiologic agents of lower respiratory tract infections.

CLINICAL MANIFESTATIONS	VIRUSES SUSPECTED	SPECIMEN COLLECTED
Upper respiratory tract infections	Influenza, parainfluenza, RSV, adenovirus, enterovirus	
Lower respiratory tract infections	Respiratory syncytial virus, parainfluenza	
CNS infections	Arbovirus, enterovirus, rabies virus, herpes virus, mumps	
Conjunctivitis	Herpes simplex virus, herpes zoster virus, adenovirus, enterovirus	
Serum hepatitis	Hepatitis B, C, D	
AIDS	Human immunodeficiency virus	
Infantile diarrhea	Rotavirus, calicivirus, Norwalk virus, astrovirus	
Parotitis	Mumps virus	
Cutaneous and mucous membrane disease	Varicella zoster virus, measles and cowpox	

Section 7: Healthcare-associated Infections (HAIs)

Healthcare-associated Infections (HAIs)

17 CHAPTER

COMPETENCY
MI8.5: Define Healthcare-associated Infections (HAIs) and enumerate types. Discuss the factors that contribute to the development of HAI and methods of prevention.
MI8.6: Describe the basics of infection control.
MI8.7: Demonstrate infection control practices and use of personal protective equipment.

HEALTHCARE-ASSOCIATED INFECTIONS (HAIs)

Definition

Infections in hospitalized patients which were not present or incubating at the time of admission. An infection acquired in a medical setting in the course of medical treatment.

- HAIs can happen in any health care facility, including hospitals, ambulatory surgical centers, end-stage renal disease facilities, and long-term care facilities.
- Bacteria, fungi, viruses, or other less common pathogens can cause HAIs.
- Prevention of nosocomial infection is the responsibility of all individuals and services provided by healthcare setting.

Major HAI Types

- Catheter associated urinary tract infections (CAUTIs)
- Central line-associated bloodstream infections (CLABSIs)
- Ventilator associated pneumonia (VAP)
- Surgical site infections (SSIs).

In a Hospital Infection Control Program runs at 2 levels:

1. ***An executive body:*** *Infection control team (ICT))*
2. ***An advisory body:*** *Infection control committee (ICC) - which adopts the legislative role of policy making.*

Functions of Hospital Infection Control Committee (HICC)

- HAI surveillance: CAUTI, CLABSI, VAP, SSI
- Develops a system for identification, reporting, analyzing and controlling HAI
- Making policies for proper antibiotic usage
- Implementing Antibiotic Stewardship Program
- Outbreak management.

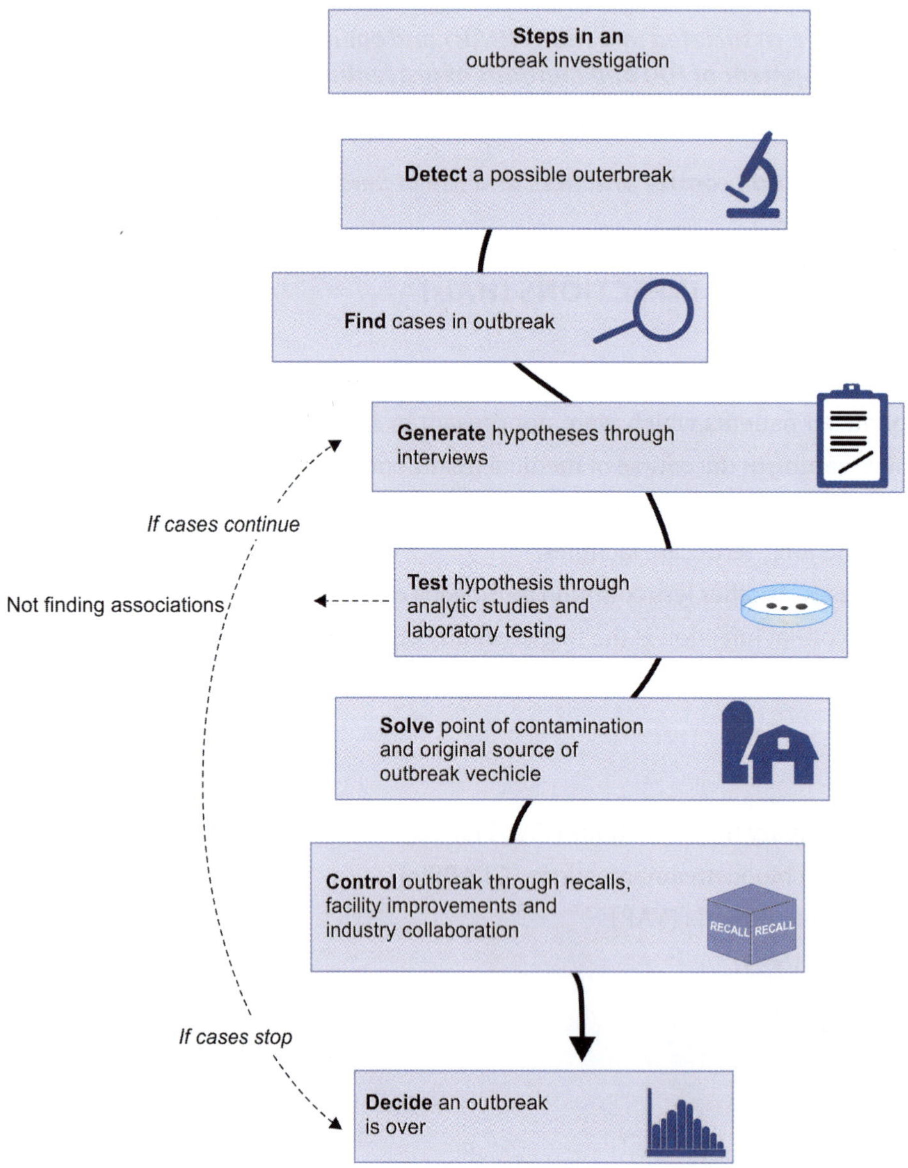

Hand Hygiene

18
CHAPTER

COMPETENCY

MI8.6: Describe the basics of infection control.

7 STEPS OF HAND WASHING

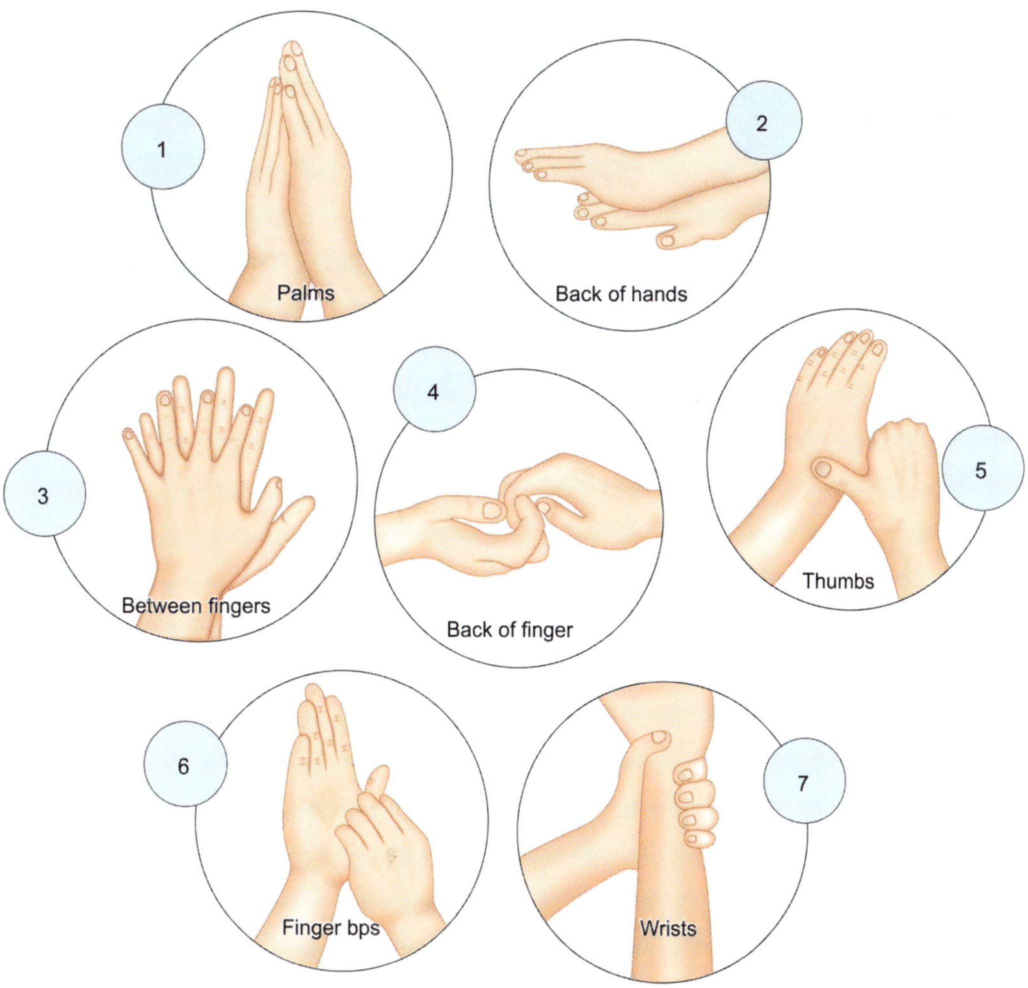

YOUR 5 MOMENTS FOR HAND HYGIENE

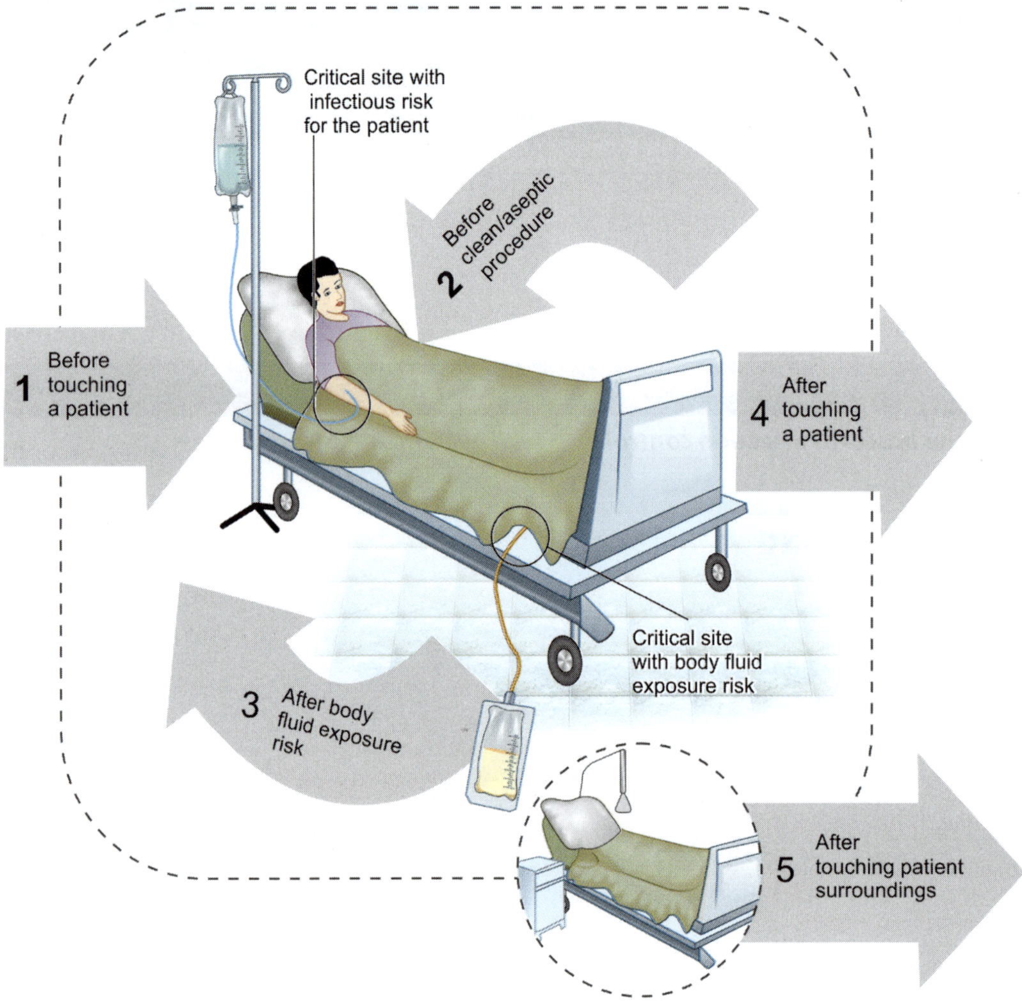

Personal Protective Equipment (PPE)

19
CHAPTER

COMPETENCY

MI8.5: Demonstrate infection control practices and use of personal protective equipment (PPE).

Sequence for PUTTING ON personal protective equipment (PPE)

The type of PPE used will vary based on the level of precautions required, such as standard and contact droplet or airborne infection isolation precautions. The procedure for putting on and removing PPE should be tailored to the specific type of PPE

1. Gown
- Fully cover torso from neck to knees, arms to end of wrists, and wrap around the back
- Fasten in back of neck and waist

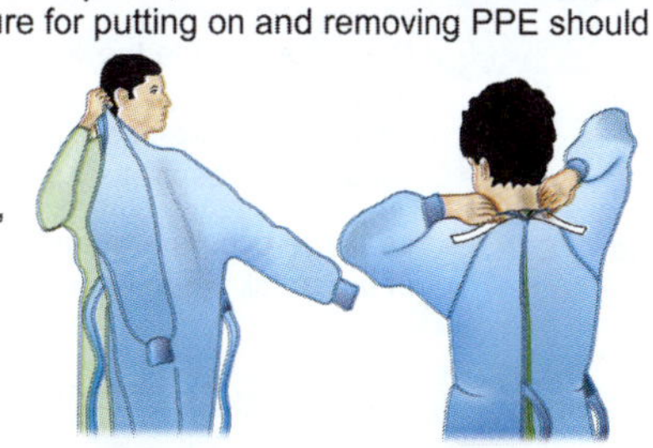

2. Mask or respirator
- Secure ties or elastic bands at middle of head and neck
- Fit flexible band to nose bridge
- Fit snug to face and below chin
- Fit-check respirator

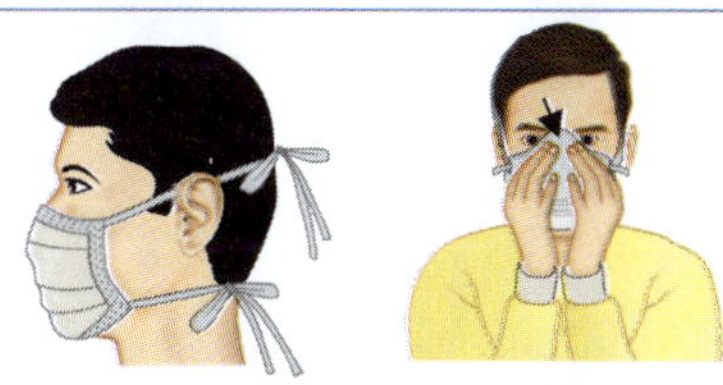

3. Goggles or face shield
- Place over face and eyes and adjust to fit

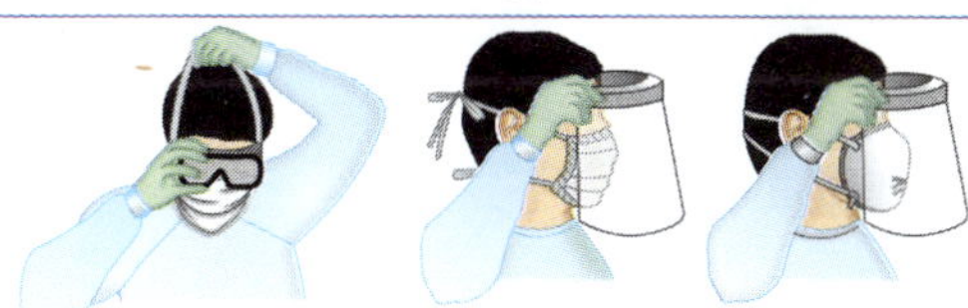

4. Gloves
- Extend to cover wrist of isolation gown

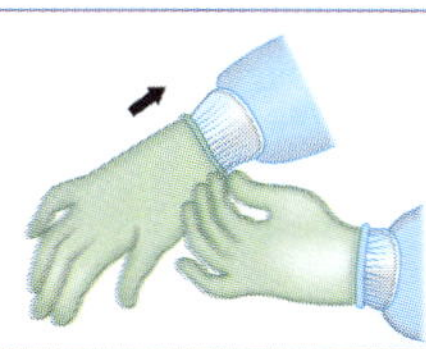

Use safe work practices to protect yourself and limit the spread of contamination
- Keep hands away from face
- Limit surfaces touched
- Change gloves when torn or heavily contaminated
- Perform hand hygiene

CDC

Understanding the difference

	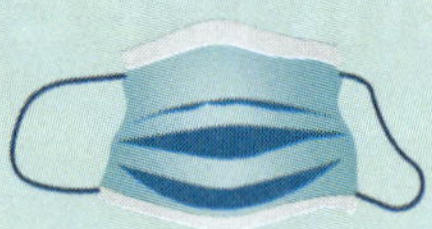 **Surgical Mask**	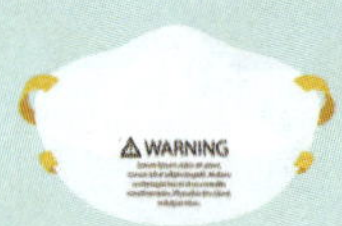 **N95 Respirator**
Testing and approval	Cleared by the U.S. food and drug administration (**FDA**)	Evaluated, tested, and approved by NIOSH as per the requirements in 42 CFR part 84
Intended use and purpose	Fluid resistant and provides the wearer protection against large droplets, splashes, or sprays of bodily or other hazardous fluids. Protects the patient from the wearer's respiratory emissions.	Reduces wearer's exposure to particles including small particle aerosois and large droplets (only non-oil aerosols)
Face seal fit	Loose-fitting	Tight-fitting
Fit testing requirement	No	Yes
User seal check requirement	No	Yes. Required each time the respirator is donned (put on)
Filtration	Does not provide the wearer with a reliable level of protection from inhaling smaller airborne particles and is not considered respiratory protection	Filters out at least 95% of airborne particles including large and small particles
Leakage	Leakage occurs around the edge of the mask when user inhales	When property fitted and donned, minimal leakage occurs around edges of the respirator when user inhales
Use limitations	Disposable, discard after each patient encounter	Ideally should be discarded after each patient encounter and after aerosol-generating procedures. It should also be discarded when it becomes damaged or deformed; no longer forms an effective seal to the face; becomes wet or visibly dirty; breathing becomes difficult; or if it becomes contaminated with blood, respiratory or nasal secretions, or other bodlly fiulds from patients

CDC NIOSH Centers for Disease Control and Prevention
National Institute for Occupational Safety and Health

Hospital Waste Management

20

CHAPTER

COMPETENCY
CM14.1: Define and classify hospital waste.
CM14.2: Describe various methods of treatment of hospital waste.
CM14.3: Describe laws related to hospital waste management.
SU15.1: Describe classification of hospital waste and appropriate methods of disposal.

Salient Features of Bio-Medical Waste Management (Amendment) Rules, 2018

1. Bio-medical waste generators including hospitals, nursing homes, clinics, dispensaries, veterinary institutions, animal houses, pathological laboratories, blood banks, healthcare facilities, and clinical establishments will have to phase out chlorinated plastic bags (excluding blood bags) and gloves by March 27, 2019.
2. All healthcare facilities shall make available the annual report on its website within a period of two years from the date of publication of the Bio-Medical Waste Management (Amendment) Rules, 2018.
3. Operators of common bio-medical waste treatment and disposal facilities shall establish bar coding and global positioning system for handling of bio-medical waste in accordance with guidelines issued by the Central Pollution Control Board by March 27, 2019.
4. The State Pollution Control Boards/ Pollution Control Committees have to compile, review and analyze the information received and send this information to the Central Pollution Control Board in a new Form (Form IV A), which seeks detailed information regarding district-wise bio-medical waste generation, information on Health Care Facilities having captive treatment facilities, information on common bio-medical waste treatment and disposal facilities.
5. Every occupier, i.e. a person having administrative control over the institution and the premises generating bio-medical waste shall pre-treat the laboratory waste, microbiological waste, blood samples, and blood bags through disinfection or sterilization on-site in the manner as prescribed by the World Health Organization (WHO) or guidelines on safe management of wastes from health care activities and WHO Blue Book 2014 and then sent to the Common bio-medical waste treatment facility for final disposal.

Bio-Medical Waste Management

Color coding instruction for segregation at the point of generation

Yellow Bag	Red Bag	Blue plastic bag/ cardboard box (puncture proof and leak proof boxes or containers with blue colored marking)	White bag (Translucent white puncture proof container)	Yellow bag (chemical and cytotoxic) C
• Anatomical waste Body tissue Organs, body parts • Soiled waste Blood and body fluid stained dressings, cotton swabs, etc. Soiled plaster casts • Discarded linen mattresses, beddings contaminated with blood or body fluid • Masks, caps, shoe cover and routine gowns • Microbiology, biotechnology and other lab waste • Blood bags (used/unused with attached tubing (labeled separate) • Discarbed medicines	Contaminated plastic waste I/V bottles, sets Tubing Catheters Syringes (without needles) Vacutainers Urine bags Gloves Disposable surgeons gowns	Glassware • Broken/discarded/ contaminated glass • Medicin evials and ampoules (except those contaminated with cytotoxic wastes) Metallic Body Implants	• Needles • Syringes with fixed needles • Scalpels • Lancets • Blades • Contaminated sharp objects that may cause punctures and cuts (including metal sharps)	• Cytotoxic drugs • Items contaminated with cytotoxic drugs along with glass or plastic ampoules, vials, etc.

Notes:

- Microbiology, biotechnology, blood bags and other laboratory waste–autoclave before disposal
- Discarded medicines shall be either sent back to manufacturer or yellow bag
- Puncture proof sharp container box to be disposed when 3/4th full or maximum
- Infected linen to be pre-treated in 1% hypochlorite
- Blue and yellow bags should be disposed within 48 hours
- Final treatment

1. Yellow bag—incineration
2. Red/White bag—autoclave
3. Blue bag—disinfection/autoclave

Section 8: Applied Exercise

Applied Exercise

21 CHAPTER

CASE STUDY 1

A 5-year-old child with fever and soreness of throat also develops difficulty in breathing. A throat swab collected is subjected to culture and a direct smear made is stained with Albert's technique. In vitro toxigenicity test also done.

A. Suggestive Organism

Corynebacterium diphtheriae, which on Albert's staining shows Chinese letter pattern/Cuneiform arrangement (V or L shaped) with metachromatic granules and greenish cytoplasm.

B. Culture Media Used

Loeffler's serum slope, Tinsdale medium and Potassium tellurite agar.

C. Clinical Manifestation of Diphtheria

- Respiratory diphtheria
- Cutaneous diphtheria
- Systemic complications.

D. Various Tests for Diphtheria Toxin Demonstration

- In vivo tests: Subcutaneous and intracutaneous tests
- In vitro tests: Elek's gel precipitation test, detection of tox gene by PCR.

E. Prophylaxis

DPT vaccine at 6,10,14 weeks given i.m.
Passive immunization - 500 to1000 units of anti-diphtheritic serum (ADS).

CASE STUDY 2

A 30-year-old female gives a history of low grade fever, cough with expectoration and mild pain in the chest since 1 year. A sputum specimen is collected for direct smear examination and for concentration and culture.

Causative Organism

Mycobacterium tuberculosis.

Morphology

On ZN staining: Red colored, straight, slightly curved rod shaped bacilli of 3×0.3 microns.

Concentration technique: Petroff's method.

Culture Medium

- Egg based (Lowenstein Jensen, Dorset, Petragnani)
- Agar based (Middlebrook 7H10 and 7H11)
- Liquid based (Middlebrook 7H12, Dubos, Proskauer and Beck, Sulas and Sauton)
- Blood based (Tarshis)
- Potato based agar (Pawlowsky).

Automated Methods

Middlebrook 7H10/7H11 available but mostly used in automated systems:

- BACTEC 460
- BACTEC MGIT 960
- SEPTI CHECK
- BacT/Alert 3D.

Clinical Features

Cough with expectoration, hemoptysis, dyspnea, fever with chills and rigor, weight loss and night sweats.

Prophylaxis

BCG is given intradermal on anterior aspect of arm.

CASE STUDY 3

A 25-year-old female with a history of having delivered at home on the previous day, is brought to Emergency room. On examination, she has a temperature of 104°F, a rapid pulse and hypotension. Blood is collected for culture and the patient is started on antibiotic therapy. The broth is inoculated on solid media. Biochemical reactions are also put up.

Condition is: Gram-negative septicemia.

Causative organism for septicemia are:

- *Gram-positive: Staphylococcus aureus, Streptococcus pyogenes, Listeria monocytogenes*
- *Gram-negative: Neisseria meningitidis, Salmonella typhi, Salmonella paratyphi A, B,* Brucella, *E. coli, Klebsiella, Proteus, Enterobacter.*

Pathogenesis of Endotoxic Shock

Lipopolysaccharide in cell wall of the gram-negative bacteria produces the shock. Inactivates monocytes, macrophages which produce TNF which induces IL-1, TNF-α. IL-1 acts on endothelial cells to produce further cytokines IL-6 and which enhances inflammatory reactions.

Endotoxic shock is characterized by fever, leukopenia, thrombocytopenia, hypotension, circulatory shock leading to death.

Laboratory Diagnosis

- Gram staining
- Blood culture on Bactec or Bac T/Alert
- Vitek-2 antimicrobial antibiotic susceptibility
- Procalcitonin
- CBC with ESR

CASE STUDY 4

A 30-year-old female comes to the out patient department complaining of curdy white discharge per vagina associated with intense pruritis. A high vaginal swab collected with aseptic precautions is subjected to culture and a smear made is stained by Gram's technique.

Causative organism: *Candida albicans.*

Culture media used: Sabouraud's dextrose agar. It can also grow on blood agar.

Gram staining: Oval budding yeast cells are seen with pseudohyphae.

Confirmatory Tests

- *Germ tube test:* Pooled human sera when mixed with a colony of *C. albicans*, kept at 37°C for 2 hours—Tube-like projections (Reynolds-Braude Phenomenon)
- Dalmau plate culture
- CHROM agar
- Sugar assimilation tests
- Immunodiagnosis: Cell wall Mannan antigen detection
- Molecular methods.

Various Lesions Caused by *Candida Albicans*

- Mucosa candidiasis: Oral thrush, vulvovaginitis, balanitis, esophageal candidiasis, angular stomatitis
- Pulmonary candidiasis
- Cutaneous candidiasis: Paronychia, intertrigo, diaper candidiasis
- Invasive candidiasis: UTI, septicemia, keratitis, keratoconjunctivitis, nosocomial.

CASE STUDY 5

A patient came from China, with history of fever and cough since 4 days and shortness of breath since 3 days. He is a known diabetic and hypertensive. Interpret the illness and how to diagnose it in current scenario.

Causative organism: *Novel Coronavirus (nCOVID-19)*

Specimen collection details:

Adapted from the WHO guidelines on 2019-nCoV.

SPECIMEN TYPE	COLLECTION MATERIALS	TRANSPORT TO LABORATORY	STORAGE TILL TESTING	COMMENT
Nasopharyngeal and oropharyngeal swab	Dacron or polyester flocked swabs	4 °C	≤ 5 days: 4 °C > 5 days: - 70 °C	The nasopharyngeal and oropharyngeal swabs should be placed in the same tube to increase the viral load
Bronchoalveolar lavage	Sterile container	4 °C	≤ 48 hours: 4 °C > 48 hours: – 70 °C	There may be some dilution of pathogen, but still a worthwhile specimen
Tracheal aspirate, nasopharyngeal aspirate or nasal wash	Sterile container	4 °C	≤ 48 hours: 4 °C > 48 hours: – 70 °C	Not applicable
Sputum	Sterile container	4 °C	≤ 48 hours: 4 °C > 48 hours: - 70 °C	Ensure the material is from the lower respiratory tract
Tissue from biopsy or autopsy including from lung	Sterile container with saline	4 °C	≤ 24 hours: 4 °C > 24 hours: – 70 °C	Autopsy sample collection preferably to be avoided
Serum (2 samples - acute and convalescent)	Serum separator tubes (adults—collect 3–5 mL whole blood)	4 °C	≤ 5 days: 4 °C > 5 days: - 70 °C	Collect paired samples: ➢ Acute—first week of illness ➢ Convalescent—2 to 3 weeks later

- ***Routine surveillance in containment zones and screening at points of entry: Choice of test (in order of priority)***
  - Rapid Antigen Test (RAT) [as per attached algorithm]
  - RT-PCR or TrueNat or CBNAAT
- ***Routine surveillance in non-containment areas: Choice of test (in order of priority)***
  - RT-PCR or TrueNat or CBNAAT
  - Rapid Antigen Test (RAT)
- ***In hospital settings: Choice of test (in order of priority)***
  - RT-PCR or TrueNat or CBNAAT
  - Rapid Antigen Test (RAT)